Supernatural Childbirth

by
Jackie Mize

Harrison House
Tulsa, Oklahoma

Unless otherwise indicated all Scripture quotations are taken from the *King James Version* of the Bible.

12 11 10 09 08   40 39 38 37 36 35 34 33 32

Supernatural Childbirth
ISBN 13: 978-0-89274-756-6
ISBN 10: 0-89274-756-0
Revised Copyright © 1995 by Jackie Mize
Copyright © 1993
P. O. Box 5788
Texarkana, TX 75505

Published by Harrison House, Inc.
P. O. Box 35035
Tulsa, Oklahoma 74153

Dedication

To Terry, my husband, the love of my life. You taught me — and sometimes made me — believe God and have faith in His Word. Because of that, we have these four great kids! Thank you for helping me receive the desires of my heart. I love you.

Contents

Foreword

by Lindsay Roberts

I praise God that Jackie has written this book on supernatural childbirth. After six pregnancies, I can say from experience that this is the greatest teaching on pregnancy and childbirth according to the Word of God that I have ever heard. Until I really discovered these spiritual principles as they apply to childbirth, I thought that I was destined for pain and problems in having babies.

I had been through two miscarriages and a tumor and very difficult times carrying a baby. When I finally carried a baby full term, I had a relatively short labor with absolutely the most incredible pain and agony I could have ever imagined. Then, after only thirty-six hours, my precious son, Richard Oral, went to be with the Lord. So after experiencing the pain of miscarriage, childbirth, and death, I certainly was open for a miracle when I became pregnant again.

I was given Jackie's tape "Supernatural Childbirth," and the title alone fascinated me. I had never heard of such a thing and my curiosity had the best of me. I needed a miracle, a supernatural intervention from God.

After listening to the entire tape, I played it over and over, taking notes on everything I heard. Immediately I began to search the Scriptures and discovered the precious truths in everything that was said. God really had redeemed me from the curse in childbirth — including pain. I continued to play the tape over and over; and I played it for my husband, my mother, and my sister-in-law and those I knew who would stand in agreement with me on God's miraculous principles of supernatural childbirth.

I was released from the bondage of fear in childbirth, especially the fear of losing another child. I learned how to speak to the baby inside me and to speak to each part of my body and command it to line up in God's perfect working order. Richard and I latched on to Bible truths about our rights in childbirth. We learned what a contraction is and what labor really is! And we were not going to let go of a word of it.

When the time came to give birth, I asked the Lord to give me a sign when it was time to go to the hospital, since I was believing for no pain. Sure enough, He did. My water broke at 10:00 p.m., and we went to the City of Faith. When I arrived they all laughed and said, "Surely you are not ready to have a baby; you're too calm, too relaxed."

So just to satisfy me, they examined me. I was already dilated to six centimeters. They hooked me up to a monitor that indicated when the contractions were coming. We all laughed because I never felt a thing! I walked and sat and talked with my family and realized that God had a miracle for me. Only toward the very end of the delivery did I experience pain. I knew immediately when I let go of God's principles and allowed my fears to take hold. I experienced about eighteen minutes of pain at the very end when I knew my precious little baby was about to be born. My mind flashed back to the past, and the devil did his best to ruin my supernatural experience.

God was victorious, though. I gave birth to the most beautiful eight pound, six ounce baby girl the world has ever seen. When our darling little Jordan Lindsay came into the world, I realized that God was totally in control of childbirth. He set the entire process up from the very beginning, and, thanks to Jackie, I experienced the birth of our little girl in the most godly, supernatural way I have ever known.

Doctors told Jackie she couldn't have babies; doctors told me I couldn't have babies. I needed to overcome fear and anxiety to be able to believe God for what His Word says: that I can have babies. It gave me great hope to see that someone had done this: Jackie had four children.

Since then we have received from the Lord two more precious little girls: Kathryn Olivia and Chloe Elizabeth. The fear that had plagued me for years that I could not have children is cast down and defeated. God surely has given us supernatural childbirth.

This divine teaching can truly change your life if you allow it to sink into your mind, body, and spirit. I pray it will richly bless you in every way as it did Richard and me.

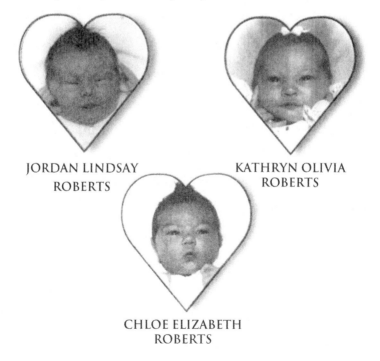

JORDAN LINDSAY ROBERTS

KATHRYN OLIVIA ROBERTS

CHLOE ELIZABETH ROBERTS

Preface

Terry and I have discovered that God has provided for every area of our life; He left nothing out. We found in the Bible that we are covenant people, that Christ has redeemed us from the curse of the law; so we keep looking in God's Word for all He has provided for us in that redemption plan.

The same way we found healing, prosperity and everything else we've ever needed from God is the same way we found God's will about children and childbirth. We studied the Bible and learned what God had to say about the situation. Then we changed what we were saying to agree with what the Bible said, what God said; in other words, we made our words agree with His Word. We found that the same laws and principles of faith we had been using in other areas would also apply to having babies.

In the area of having babies, there have certainly been many things said over the years – some good and some bad, some right and some wrong. Most things told to us are from someone's experience, and it was usually bad. Pregnancy, as the world views it, is nine months of misery. People laugh and joke about it. They expect a pregnant woman to get depressed, to be moody and blue, to miss her mother and hate her husband: to be an overall basket case for nine months. It's supposed to be a terrible experience for the husband. He feels as though he should walk on egg shells trying to keep his wife happy because she is sick to her stomach, has morning sickness, craves pickles and ice cream and hates sex. All in all, it's not a pretty picture and certainly not a pleasant experience.

Delivery, or birth, the world says, should be equally a disaster. Every movie or television program that shows a woman giving birth confirms the horror stories that have been handed down for generations from friends and relatives. Women are told that it has to take twelve to twenty hours of pain and agony, and they will think they are dying. They are told it is the most horrible pain in the world…. Heard enough?

Boy, I have! Unfortunately, this picture was about all I had seen or heard on this subject, and I'm sure the same is probably true for you.

But Terry and I decided a long time ago that we wanted to know what God has to say about every area of our lives. We have sound, fundamental belief that God is smarter than we are and smarter than anyone else as well. So we have to find out what He says and then learn to make it work in our real life situation.

In this book I want to share with you some truths that Terry and I have learned from God's Word and how we put them into use. They've been a blessing to us. They have totally changed the course of our lives, and we want them to help you change and accomplish what needs to be done in your life.

We have shared these truths with people all over the world and people have received tremendous miracles in their lives because they received what God has to say about having children.

I pray that you'll open your heart to receive what the Spirit of God has to say to you. I pray that when you finish this book you'll have a greater confidence in God and in your covenant with Him, and faith will have risen in your heart for your own circumstances, whatever they might be.

Introduction

To Jackie and me the words "supernatural childbirth" aren't just a catchy phrase or a sermon title. These words to us mean Lynn, Paul, Lori and Cristy. Supernatural childbirth to us means faith in God's Word to bring about what man has declared impossible.

When Jackie and I met and began talking marriage, she said to me, "If we are going to get married, there is something about me you should know."

"I CAN'T HAVE CHILDREN!" she said.

What a devastating statement! Women around the world have made the same declaration. My question to them now is the same question I posed to Jackie over two decades ago. "Oh, really? Who said? Who said you can't have children?" It makes a major difference in every area of your life, who said. I am always asking people that question, "Who said?"

Jackie answered me, "The doctors said."

"Oh, I see. Well, God said you can have babies," I told her. "Even though I thank God for doctors and hospitals, and medical science is always advancing, they are not our source, our final authority; God is, and God said you can have children."

"He did?"

"Sure. The Bible is full of Scriptures about children. He said He makes the barren woman to keep house and be a joyful mother of children. He said your children will be as olive plants and your wife as a fruitful vine. The Bible says there will be neither male nor female barren among God's people. We will have all the children we want."

And we did. We have four children — two boys and two girls. And we've taken them around the world with us giving Living Bread to dying men, sharing the gospel with the world that cost the blood of Jesus.

Jackie's testimony of supernatural childbirth has gone literally around the world. In many nations where I go, people come up to me and say, "I've heard your wife's tape on supernatural childbirth." We have files of testimonies from women at home and abroad who have beautiful children because they applied these faith principles from God's Word. That is what Jackie is sharing here in this long requested and long awaited book — faith principles, faith principles from the Bible that will work for you in any area of your life. We strongly believe that any man, woman, boy or girl can take God's Word and change his/her circumstances through faith and prayer.

Something that Jackie and I want people to understand is that to us, supernatural childbirth is being able to believe God to get pregnant, carry that baby to full term, and have a healthy mommy deliver a healthy baby. Many people think that supernatural childbirth only means having painless childbirth because that is what Jackie did with three of our four children; but we've never been dogmatic about that. Our point is having the baby and being healthy. The painless part and all the other extras we've had and believed for are available for you as you use your faith and "shoot for the stars; go for the best; aim high!" Those are faith principles. With God and faith you can always go all out and aim high. The bottom line is this: the Bible says, "According to your faith." There isn't a right way and a wrong way in this book. There isn't "Jackie's way." It's according to your faith. We got what we used our faith for. We believe you will too!

For the only cause that counts

— world harvest,

Terry L. Mize

1

Where Do You Start?

When Terry and I got married, May 10, 1969, we had so many things that looked like they were working against us. The doctor had told me for years that I'd never be able to have a baby at all — that I couldn't carry one. He said, "If by some slim chance you were ever to get pregnant, you'd have to spend the whole nine months in bed. But, even at that, I doubt that you could carry it." Well-meaning friends of the family and family members all said to Terry, "You know, Jackie can't have children. It's really a shame too, the way she loves babies and has always wanted to have a house full."

We didn't know the Word then like we do now, but Terry did know that God healed and he knew some basics of the Bible from growing up in church. He knew we could pray and change things. Most of all, he knew God and knew that God's Word was always, and in every area, accurate. For all the years I've known him, his standard comment on any subject is "Who said?" It makes a big difference who said it. "What does God say? What does the Bible say?" So he told me, "I appreciate medical doctors and medical science. They've come a long way, and I hope they go farther. But they are not our source, our answer, our final authority. God says we can have children. We'll have all the children we want."

We didn't know the details or the methods or exactly how to make it work in those early days, but we knew the will of God was to have children. It was His idea; He thought children up. He ordered them in the Garden of Eden. We knew that we could, that we would, have babies.

We prayed and we were so excited to find out, after we were married only a few months, that I was expecting our first baby. Even though all the things I had been told about not being able to have babies were all so real in my mind, and of course, had produced so many fears, I did have hope because we had prayed and asked God for children. Terry had just about convinced me it was possible, and I began to have faith in his faith that God would answer our prayer.

When I was about eight weeks along, I started bleeding, and all the fears and doubts I had came back. Within a few hours, I lost the baby.

Even though I was only a few weeks pregnant, that baby was as real to me as any baby I had ever seen. Any woman who has been pregnant knows what I'm talking about too. Many times men don't understand the trauma of a miscarriage because to them the baby is not a reality yet. They often try to comfort their wife with, "It's okay — we will try again." And that doesn't comfort us, because to a woman that baby is a reality from conception. It affects mothers because it is not just a "miscarriage"; it is the loss of a child. And it takes a period of time to recover emotionally, just as it does with the loss of any loved one.

Of course, the fears, anxieties and everything terrible that everyone had told me still bombarded my mind. It looked like it was just impossible for us to ever have children, and to have children was the desire of my heart. I had no greater ambition (and still don't) than to be a wife and mother. I was convinced that was the very best job I could ever have in the whole world — and you know what? It is. I've made the statement for years that to be Terry's wife and our four children's mother is the highest calling I could ever achieve.

For a whole year, I cried each month when my period came because I wanted to be pregnant and wasn't.

Then Terry got drafted into the army, and we moved three hundred miles away from everyone we knew and everyone who knew us. That was very good for us. We were on our own. We spent serious time getting into the Word of God and building our faith.

We decided to pray and ask God for a baby. We prayed and believed God that we would have a baby, and I got pregnant again. This time we knew, that we knew, that we knew, that we would have a baby. We did everything that we wanted to do. Terry was stationed at Ft. Bliss in El Paso, Texas, and we didn't have a car, so we rode a borrowed motorcycle until I was so big with the baby that I was embarrassed to ride it anymore. We did everything. We even went mountain climbing outside of El Paso. And not one time did I even start to miscarry. You see, once we made up our minds and determined in our hearts that we were going to have a baby, that we could pray, that God would hear and answer that prayer because it was His will, that's what God did. God will meet you at your level of faith — whatever that level is — and that's where our faith was.

Terry was in the army, and they do things a little differently in the army. They put me in the hospital a few days before the baby was even due because they thought he was going to be a large baby and they wanted to watch me. The doctors said because of possible complications, they were going to induce labor Wednesday morning, August 11, 1971.

Well, we knew that we could pray and God would hear our prayer. It was no big faith feat — we didn't know anything about faith — we just knew the simple truth that God would hear our prayers. We have always believed that prayer changes things. We prayed that I'd go into labor by myself — that labor would not be induced — that the baby would be born before noon, and that the labor would be short. (We didn't know at that time we could pray for a painless delivery.) It was stretching our faith to believe to deliver the baby safe and whole, in a short time.

The hospital staff got real busy and didn't have time to induce me into labor. I went into labor by myself, and after three hours and fifteen minutes, our little miracle, that the doctors said would never happen, arrived. Lynn Noel, not a large baby — only seven pounds, five ounces — was born at 11:45 a.m. on the very day he was due, just as we prayed. We got everything we prayed for.

Because I was a gestation diabetic (diabetes showing only during pregnancy), we were depending on God to balance Lynn's blood sugar. Being in an army hospital, procedures were done routinely. They immediately began an intravenous solution of sugar water in the veins of my baby's tiny little head so the insulin would not cause him to convulse. It was awful the first time Terry and I saw Lynn with needles taped to the sides of his shaved little head. But in only a few hours, his blood sugar level had come into balance, and we never had another problem with it.

Before I got pregnant again, we applied our faith against diabetes and declared, "I'm healed by the stripes of Jesus." In the next three pregnancies, I always made it a point to tell the doctors that I had been a gestation diabetic and should be checked. The tests always came back negative. Diabetes was never a factor again.

The world has programmed women to expect a long, torturous delivery with their first baby. But it doesn't have to be that way for those who have a covenant with God.

We have to totally change our thinking by renewing our mind with the Word of God on the subject of having babies, the same way we renew our mind concerning finances,

health, and everything else. We can no longer think the way
the world thinks if we want to have the results, the promises
and provisions that have been given to us as born-again
believers. We have to find out what God thinks on any
subject and begin to think and talk the way He does.
Romans 12:2 says,

**And be not conformed to this world: but be ye
transformed by the renewing of your mind, that ye may
prove what is that good, and acceptable, and perfect,
will of God.**

Supernatural vs. Natural

After we had Lynn, and we got out of the army, we
went into the ministry and moved to Mexico as
missionaries. We grew in faith as we spent time studying
the Bible and listening to tapes. We saw God do mighty
miracles in our lives and in the ministry. We traveled all the
time, and although I really wanted another baby soon, I
didn't think it could be worked in at that point since we
weren't settled in one place.

We came back to the United States for the holidays and
attended a meeting that changed our lives. (Keep in mind
now that I had had one miscarriage and our baby, Lynn,
was about two years old.) It was one of Kenneth Copeland's
"Super Sunday" meetings. Brother Copeland finished
teaching his message and then began to prophesy. "The
Lord says, 'There are ladies in here now who are expecting
a baby and others who want to have babies. If you'll use My
Word and stand on My Word, you'll have those babies
supernaturally without pain. The doctors and nurses and
medical personnel will be astounded and amazed at the
way you come through this delivery. It will be something
they haven't seen before. And after they see with their
medical eyes what you have done — that yes, it is true, they
have witnessed it — then you can tell them that God did it.

It will be a testimony to them.'"

Well, that just went off on the inside of both Terry and me. We knew it was the truth; it was possible! This was one of those times that you hear something the very first time and you know without a shadow of a doubt that it's right, but you don't understand how in the world it will happen.

I want to clarify the difference between what I am calling "supernatural" childbirth and what everyone else calls "natural" childbirth. In natural childbirth classes there are exercises. The woman is taught to center in on a focal point, to pant and breathe as directed, and the husband is taught to coach her through it, and so forth. This method does work to a degree and praise God for it! Without it, many women would have had really bad experiences in giving birth. Natural childbirth is good, but God always has a better way of doing everything. Supernatural always exceeds natural in any area. And when we decide to do it His way, the results are amazing!

When I refer to supernatural childbirth, I'm talking strictly about being able to conceive and to have babies with a pregnancy free from nausea, morning sickness, pain, moodiness, depression and without fear of any kind; then going through the entire labor without pain, and through the delivery without stitches and anesthetic. I'm talking about using the Word of God to overcome, change and make things better.

When we heard those words in Brother Copeland's meeting, I could not imagine how it would work. I didn't know anyone in the whole world who had done it or even thought it was possible. So we were facing something that we knew absolutely nothing about. But we knew when it went off in our spirit, "This is for us!" The Bible says children are the heritage of the Lord, a blessing. (Ps. 127:3.) They can start off being a blessing and continue being a blessing right on through life. We studied in the Word and the more we studied, the more we knew that was true. So we started believing God right then that we would have our next baby without fear, pain or problems.

We returned to Guadalajara, Mexico, as missionaries; and in a few months, I found out I was pregnant.

At that time, I didn't know anybody in the whole world who had ever had a baby without thinking they were dying. When I had Lynn, I thought I was dying. It was terrible. I was so afraid. It sounds so easy to say, "I went to the hospital and had a baby," but any woman who has done it knows there is a lot of hard work involved. And I was scared. I thank God the labor lasted only three hours and fifteen minutes; but I was scared that whole time, and I didn't know how to handle that fear.

I knew in my heart now that there was a way to have a baby without pain and without fear. Of course, my head told me many reasons it wouldn't work, but we were growing in the Word and refused to allow the devil to steal this truth from us. We continuously made our words agree with God's Word, listened to good, faith-building tapes, prayed and read the Bible.

2

What Does God Say?

Terry and I began studying the Bible on the subject of conception, pregnancy and child rearing. We found that the first spoken words of God, the Creator, to man, the creature, was about having a family. **Be fruitful, and multiply, and replenish the earth** (Gen. 1:28). Having a family was God's idea; God thought up having babies. So where did the "sorrow" in childbirth come from?

Originally it came on Adam and Eve in the Garden of Eden. (See "Epilogue.")

> **Unto the woman he said, I will greatly multiply thy sorrow and thy conception; in SORROW thou shalt bring forth children; and thy desire shall be to thy husband, and he shall rule over thee.**
>
> **Genesis 3:16**

If the end of the story was that since man sinned the curse came on him and the earth, then there would be no hope. But, thank God, at that same time God promised a Savior to us. **And I will put enmity between thee and the woman, and between thy seed and her seed; it shall bruise thy head, and thou shalt bruise his heel** (Gen. 3:15). And Jesus did come and redeem us.

> **Christ hath redeemed us from the curse of the law, being made a curse for us: for it is written, Cursed is every one that hangeth on a tree.**
>
> **Galatians 3:13**

> **Surely he hath borne our GRIEFS, and carried our sorrows: yet we did esteem him stricken, smitten of God, and afflicted.**

But he was wounded for our transgressions, he was bruised for our iniquities: the chastisement of our peace was upon him; and with his stripes we are healed.
Isaiah 53:4,5

It is interesting to me that the word translated "griefs" in Isaiah 53:4 has the same meaning as the word translated "sorrow" in Genesis 3:16. That's as plain as it can be. Jesus bore that sorrow, that grief, so that we don't have to. Isn't that good news? I don't have to bear sorrow and grief!

We believe He redeemed us from sin, sickness and poverty. "By His stripes we are healed." If that healing delivers us from pain, then that's what it does. It doesn't matter if the pain comes in the form of cancer, migraine headaches, stomach aches or childbearing. If we're redeemed, we're redeemed; either we are or we're not! And I believe we are!

Some people have told Terry and me, "Well, I don't believe that." I won't argue about it with anyone. I am just telling you we saw it in the Bible, and we made it work for us with our last three children. If it will work for us, it will work for you. The reason it worked for us is we found it in God's Word and kept reading, studying and talking it until it was part of us. And that's what will make it work for you.

We were driving on a trip one day, and I was reading the Bible out loud to Terry, as I do many times. I just opened the Bible to the book of Exodus and began to read. Terry said, "Read that again." I did. He said, "Read it again." So I did. We began to get really excited as we saw that Hebrew women had their babies differently than the Egyptian women. We saw in Exodus how the Hebrew women, even in captivity in Egypt, knew Abraham's covenant and walked in its blessings.

And the king of Egypt spake to the Hebrew midwives, of which the name of the one was Shiphrah, and the name of the other Puah:

And he said, When ye do the office of a midwife to the Hebrew women, and see them upon the stools; if it be a son, then ye shall kill him: but if it be a daughter, then she shall live.

But the midwives feared God, and did not as the king of Egypt commanded them, but saved the men children alive.

And the king of Egypt called for the midwives, and said unto them, Why have ye done this thing, and have saved the men children alive?

And the midwives said unto Pharaoh, Because the Hebrew women are not as the Egyptian women; FOR THEY ARE LIVELY, and are delivered ere the midwives come in unto them.

Exodus 1:15-19

It said, **The Hebrew women are not as the Egyptian women**. The women with a covenant are not like the women without a covenant. These Hebrew women knew and acted on their covenant and had their babies fast and easily. Many people have thought that those midwives were just lying about that situation, but they weren't. Those Hebrew women knew their covenant. And the apostle Paul said we have an even better covenant today. (Heb. 8:6.)

That the blessing of Abraham might come on the Gentiles through Jesus Christ; that we might receive the promise of the Spirit through faith...

And if ye be Christ's, then are ye Abraham's seed, and heirs according to the promise.

Galatians 3:14,29

We found in 1 Timothy 2:15, **Notwithstanding she shall be saved in childbearing, if they continue in faith and charity and holiness with sobriety.** That word "saved" means kept safe and sound. Isn't that good to be kept safe and sound in childbirth? That's comforting to me.

We were excited as we began to see these things in the Word of God, but we didn't share them with anyone. We had never heard of anyone else doing this before, and we didn't need anyone's unbelief or doubt. We didn't need anyone arguing with us and telling us it wouldn't work. I had enough to do just keeping out all the doubt, unbelief and fear that came against my mind; I certainly didn't want to invite any from other people. So we didn't tell anyone about it. As long as I told myself, God and the devil, we decided those were the only ones who needed to know. We set ourselves in agreement with the Bible, and I would declare to Terry what I was believing, and he would agree with me. Then Terry would make those same declarations back to me. We both would be saying them and hearing them. And, of course, faith grew. But my head still screamed at me, "You've got to be kidding — this can't happen; it's impossible." I thank God that we learned that even if you can't out think the devil, you can out talk him by saying what God says.

Get in Agreement

At that time I relied on Terry and his faith a lot to carry me through in some areas. Now Terry didn't say to me, "Bless God, you're going to do it this way, and that's all there is to it." He said, "I am going to agree with you at whatever level your faith is; wherever you are, I'm with you. I'll read the Word to you and believe with you and help you however I can; but since I'm not the one who is going to have the baby, it is going to have to be done with your faith."

I know there are times a wife doesn't have her husband in agreement with her. But I believe she can set herself in agreement with God's Word, and God will honor her faith and bring it to pass.

On the other hand, it doesn't matter how spiritual, how great, how wonderful a husband is, he is not going into the delivery room and have that baby himself. When it gets down to the nitty-gritty, it is the woman who is going to have that baby. It is going to be her faith that comes through. So husbands, the best thing you can do is come into agreement with your wife. If you get into disagreement, the Word of God won't work for you. How can two walk together unless they be agreed? (Amos 3:3.) Encourage her, read the Bible to her (faith comes by hearing, Rom.10:17), then find out where her faith is, and come into agreement with her. Then you will see results.

I learned to grow in the confidence that it really would work. I was Abraham's seed, and I had been redeemed. I continued to study the Bible and say what God said about my children, body — everything. And I grew in faith.

3

How Does It Work?

Our first baby, Lynn, was now past two years old. As I said, I had carried him full term and delivered him in a little over three hours. But still I was really ignorant of the details of the process of childbirth — how your body changes, what all has to happen — so I made it a point to read every book I could get on the subject. The unknown produces fear. I realized that the more knowledge I had of what my body had to do, the less likely I was to be afraid. Once I understood what was happening as changes took place in my body, I was no longer afraid. The more knowledge I gained, the more peace and confidence I had. Of course, there are usually a few things in every good source of information that you have to toss out because it doesn't agree with what you are believing for. For example, most books tell you to expect a long labor with your first baby and severe afterbirth pains after your second baby. I heard someone say, "You should have as much sense as an old cow: eat the hay and spit out the sticks." I always tried to keep that in mind as I read those books. The more knowledge you have about what's going on inside of you, the better off you are. Just always spit out the sticks.

One major thing I realized was that I was going to have to watch what I said. If I was believing God that I would have this baby without pain, then I would have to quit expecting and talking about labor pains. (People always say, "How far apart are the labor pains?") I wondered, *What should I call them? I refuse to call them pains.* And then I remembered the nurse called them contractions. So that's what I called them from then on: muscle contractions.

Sometimes people get silly ideas, and I was no different. I couldn't imagine how you could have a baby without hurting. I thought, *Would you just not know what was going on?* I wondered, *Will I just wake up and there will be a baby in bed with me? I mean, how will I know?*

God took me step by step. I asked Him about everything. I said, "God, I don't understand how this is going to happen. I've already had one baby, and I know all the things that happened and that it was hard work, but I don't understand how my body will contract and stretch without hurting."

I knew labor "pains" were muscle contractions, but I didn't understand why they *did* hurt so I didn't understand why they *wouldn't* hurt. It didn't make sense to me. The Lord explained it so plainly that I couldn't miss it. "Contract the muscle in your arm," He said. I did.

"Now hold it." I did. I held it real tight. "Keep holding it. Hold it for as long as you can." I did. My arm was all tensed up, and the muscle was tight; it was hard, and it began to tremble, but it didn't hurt.

He said, "That is a muscle contraction, and it doesn't have to hurt." It was uncomfortable and a strain on my muscles, but it didn't hurt.

That changed my whole way of thinking. It explained to me how it could work. I knew that in order to push the baby out the muscles had to contract. The Lord explained to me, "When your body goes into labor, the contractions will come. Your body will work hard as the muscles contract. They'll push the baby and cause everything to do what it should, but it doesn't have to hurt." The pain women experience in childbirth comes mostly from fear and lack of knowledge. This keeps them from being able to stay in control of the situation and keeps them from having the peace of God during labor and delivery. Pain came when

Adam and Eve had to leave the Garden because of sin. Pain is under the curse. ALL pain — headache, stomach pain, toothache — is under the curse.

Since Jesus has redeemed us from pain, we don't have to put up with it. It's up to us whether we take authority over pain and run it off in Jesus' name or we let it stay. The choice is ours.

How Will I Know When It's Time?

I really didn't know my baby's due date because before I got pregnant this time, God had miraculously healed me from a tumor. My closest estimate was sometime between the first week of August and the first week of October.

Since we were missionaries and our home was Guadalajara, Mexico, we decided that I would stay there to have the baby rather than come back to the United States like everyone suggested. God gave me a wonderful Spirit-filled doctor, we found a good hospital and my mother came down for the big event.

Even though my doctor was a Christian, I didn't tell him what we were believing to have happen or not to happen during this birth because I didn't want to take a chance that he might try to talk me out of it. But I did tell him I wouldn't need any anesthetic.

One day at the end of August, I started having light contractions. I knew the labor was going to be fast, and I knew it was going to be easy, so I just kept wondering all day if this was it. I would have a contraction about every two or three hours, so I decided to go to the doctor and have him check me. He said, "Don't even go all the way out to your house tonight. The baby weighs at least seven pounds, and you've already started dilating. You'll have that baby before the night is over."

Well, that night came and went, and many other nights came and went. I had no more contractions. Six weeks later I was still pregnant, and I was getting so big, I could hardly get up out of a chair or take a deep breath. The baby was taking up every available space I had and was still growing! I knew he was bigger than Lynn had been. I was beginning to think I was eternally pregnant!

Finally I figured up and said to Terry, "I know without a doubt this baby has to be due. Yesterday was the last possible due date I could have had — October 5. This baby is at least one day past due."

I didn't ever want to have a baby early. God knew what He was doing, and nine months is how long it takes for a baby to be strong, fully developed and ready to be born. I never wanted to try to believe God to speed things up or have a baby born at a more convenient time. But I must admit, those six weeks were the longest six weeks I have ever spent in my life, thinking each day would be "it."

That night, Terry and I sat down on the bed and opened the Bible. Terry said, "The Lord just spoke to me and told me to mirror His Word to Him." In other words, tell Him what His Word says. "So that's what I'm going to do, and then we're going to pray."

We started in Genesis where the curse came on Adam and Eve. Then we went to Galatians 3:14,29 where it shows us we've been redeemed from the curse. We read the curses in Deuteronomy 28 and said, "No, we'll not have that; we are redeemed from the curse." We went to Mark 11:23,24 that tells us we can have what we say. We read Matthew 18:19 that talks about the prayer of agreement. We read 1 Timothy 2:15 that says a woman will be saved in childbearing. We told God what we were believing. We said, "God, this is what You said in Your Word. This is what we believe. This is what we've been standing on. This is what we've been confessing that we will have."

Then Terry said, "Devil, I want you and all hell to listen. This is what we are believing, and we'll have nothing less than this. Jackie will go to the hospital and have this baby without pain, without stitches, without anesthetic, without any complications, without any problems."

We called God and all of heaven to record on what God had said; and then we wanted the devil and all of hell to know what God had said and where we stood in this matter.

Then Terry laid his hands on my large round abdomen and said, "Body, you function perfectly, the way you should function to have a baby. Bones, joints, you spread where you need to spread. Muscles, you contract the way you need to contract. Cervix, you soften and dilate fast, easily, without problems. Vagina, you stretch easily; you be elastic and stretch perfectly without tearing." He spoke to every part of my body that we could think of.

We said, "This is our last night of this pregnancy. Our baby will be born in the morning."

Then he spoke to the baby. "Baby, I command you in the name of Jesus Christ of Nazareth to get in position and to be born in the morning." It was already past midnight then, so Terry went on to pray that I would have a good night's sleep, rest well and wake up refreshed and ready to go to the hospital to have the baby.

Speak to everything you can think of, then be confident that your body and your baby have to line up and obey the name of Jesus.

Now we had a small dilemma: since we had never known anyone who had done this, we really didn't know what to expect. Finally we decided that we would command my water to break. Thank God! We could at least have a sign, something so we would know I was in labor and should go to the hospital.

I took a shower, got my things ready to go to the hospital and went to bed. At this stage in pregnancy a good night's rest was welcomed. I had slept soundly for about five hours when the baby dropped into position, jarring me awake. I had never experienced anything like it, but I knew what had happened, so I got up and went into the bathroom. One little trickle of water ran down my leg. I didn't know if my water broke or if it was just pressure on my bladder. (The doctor broke my water when Lynn was born so I didn't know what to expect.) I thought, *There's got to be more than this to be sure, Lord. I still don't know if it's time.*

I went back to bed for an hour; and when I got up again, I left a small puddle of water with every step I took. This was it! I had my first contraction. It was so intense that I was surprised. I realized that if they started out like that, it wouldn't take very many of them to have that baby. They came at five minute intervals. After about four or five of them, I woke Terry and said, "You'd better get up. This is it."

Beginning with the first contraction, every muscle was working, contracting and pushing, but without pain. The contractions were so intense that if I were walking when one started, I would have to stop and wait until it passed to take another step, but they didn't hurt! *I can remember thinking, I know this is the way God intended for women to have babies from the beginning.*

On the way to the hospital there was one contraction that was even more intense. I thought the baby was going to be born in the car before we reached the hospital and that scared me. And because I became fearful, the next contraction really hurt bad. I knew I had to gain control fast. I said, "Terry, pray for me. That one scared me and hurt." He reached his hand over and laid it on my abdomen and said, "We're not going to have any fear or pain. Go in Jesus' name."

Terry told me, "Jackie, I can't believe this for you. We're in this together; we're believing together. But it is up to you once you get in that hospital room. If you decide you want to have an anesthetic or something for pain, just know, I'm in agreement with you no matter what you do." I had a decision to make: either go ahead and make this work like we said and believed it would or give in, quit using my faith and take whatever came. I remember after Terry prayed for me in the car I stomped my foot and said, "Devil, I refuse to hurt and be afraid." By the time I had the next contraction, we had won. I was back in faith and peace instead of fear. All pain was gone. I am sure that was where I made up my mind and became absolutely determined to run the devil off and take what was rightfully mine.

When we finally got to the hospital, it was almost funny. The nurses asked, "Can we help you?"

"I'm going to have a baby," I told them.

"We can see that," they replied.

I told them, "I mean right now!" They didn't believe me, because I was just standing there at the counter and smiling and talking normally.

The contractions were about one-and-one-half minutes apart and were lasting about that long. Since we were in Mexico and I was still having a challenge learning the language, we were talking through an interpreter. It was really fun trying to convince the interpreter to convince the nurses to hurry.

I told them, "I'll give you ten minutes and that's all the time you've got to get ready." They all laughed. They didn't believe I was even close to time for delivery.

We finally convinced them to examine me, and when they did, they realized I was right. I was completely dilated. But I missed it on the time: it was twenty minutes until the baby was born, not ten. But my sweet Christian doctor got there a little late; he arrived just in time to hear the baby cry.

It was the most wonderful thing I had ever experienced because I didn't have fear. I had confidence and peace instead. I experienced a joy and a thrill that no words could ever express as I gave that one big push to get that second miracle baby out and into the hands of a Mexican doctor I didn't even know.

From the beginning of labor to the time our baby Paul David was born was only forty minutes. He weighed a hearty ten pounds — which I could hardly believe. I told God, "I would have agreed that Your Word worked if I would have had a six-pound baby. And people would have been amazed if I would have had a six-pound baby with only forty minutes in labor, without pain and without stitches and without complications. That would have been a wonderful testimony. But a ten-pound baby! Only You would do that!" (I was glad I didn't know how big the baby was before I had him!)

It's Not Over Yet!

The very next thing that presented itself was, "Since this is your second baby, you will have afterbirth pains, and they are really bad. In fact, they are worse than the labor pains."

Let me tell you, those afterbirth pains are under the same curse as any other pain. After you have your baby, keep talking to your body, keep telling it what to do. It is subject to you; you are not subject to your body. You can use the name of Jesus and make your body do what it needs to. Command the bleeding to stop. Command the uterus to contract like it is supposed to, without pain. It is still only a contraction and does not have to hurt.

The doctors and nurses had never seen anything like it. They had never seen anybody walk into the hospital laughing, lie down on the delivery table, push once, have a ten-pound baby and an hour later call friends and family in the United States announcing the baby. I never felt better in my life.

4

What Should I Say?

Many people think they have to tell the doctors, hospital staff, relatives, and everyone they see just what they believe.

My doctor in Mexico was Spirit-filled and attended the church we were involved with there in Guadalajara, but we didn't tell him exactly what we were believing for. He respected Terry — he knew he was a man of God — so it was easy for him to go along with us in the things we did tell him.

When the nurses asked me about an anesthetic I said, "I won't need any." They looked at me like I was a little strange, but they said, "We'll have it here, and if you need it, you can ask for it." I said, "That's fine with me." That way it didn't disturb them; but yet, I had the baby and never needed any anesthetic. (I didn't feel that it hurt my faith at all since the anesthetic was there for them and not for me.) That made an impression. They could accept it because they saw me do it, not because they heard me make some wild confession about what all I was going to do.

You need to make your confessions out loud first to yourself (and to your husband if he is in agreement) because faith comes by hearing. Second, confess it to God because you are reminding Him, as well as yourself, what He has said in His Word. And then third, tell the devil, because you certainly want him to know where you stand and that you're not going to budge an inch. No one else needs to know.

Don't make the mistake of telling everyone what you're believing. It is enough to deal with the doubt and unbelief that come against your mind from the devil without having to answer to relatives and friends too: "Why doesn't it look like it's working? Why hasn't anyone else ever done this?"

People have asked me, "What did you tell your doctor, the nurses, the personnel in the delivery room?" Nothing. It was none of their business what I was doing.

When you go into the hospital, that's not the time to have all your confession cards out, yelling and screaming with every contraction. "Bless God, I'm going to have this baby without pain." It's too late. If you haven't built up a confidence on the inside of you by then and you are in pain, tell them to give you a shot so you can relax. You don't have to impress anybody. You don't have to try to prove God is God. You don't have to wave your Bible and tell them what a great spiritual person you are. If you walk in with confidence and peace and say, "I'm going to have my baby now," they'll work with you. They'll do everything they can to help you when you cooperate with them.

But when a woman walks in the hospital like some kind of a religious weirdo, that's exactly what they will think she is. Then that gives a bad testimony of what a Christian is because many times the lady isn't really in faith and what she is screaming and confessing doesn't happen. Faith is having confidence, being totally at peace — confident that it is all working. **And this is the confidence that we have in him, that, if we ask any thing according to his will, he heareth us** (1 John 5:14).

When you go to the hospital, you can quietly make your confessions, your declarations, if you want to. You can talk to your body if you want to. But when the nurse comes into the labor room, you don't have to slap her in the face with your confessions. You don't have to hide anything, but you can be discreet — just be in control. Do what you need to do to stay in control, but still be kind and act in love to everyone there. Sometimes that speaks the loudest and is one of the best testimonies we can have as a Christian.

Let Them SEE the Difference

We were living in the United States when I had my third baby — my second one supernaturally. During the entire last two months of my pregnancy the doctor said I would deliver the baby early. We declared that we had tithers' rights. I would not have a baby prematurely because we paid our tithes. (Mal. 3:10.) And I didn't. In fact, when the doctor decided I was two weeks past my due date, he scheduled me to go to the hospital and be induced into labor. That morning, as Terry took me to the hospital, we continued to believe I would go into labor on my own. When we got to the hospital, I was laughing and talking. The nurse was the sweetest one I'd ever had. She took me into the labor room, but before they could induce me, I began to have contractions, so all they did was break my water.

When the nurse came back into the labor room she said, "I'm not even going to check you. It's going to be a while before you do anything."

I said, "I wouldn't be too sure about that."

"Now honey," she said, "your smile has to change, and your smile hasn't changed yet, so it's still going to be a while. You'll be here until way after noon." (That was at 10:30 a.m.)

"Don't go off too far," I kidded her, "because when I call for you, you'd better get here. I know what I'm talking about. This won't take all day. I have my babies fast." She laughed and went on.

In less than thirty minutes I started having the urge to push. Terry got the nurse, and when she checked me, I was fully dilated and ready to go to the delivery room. She got all excited and could hardly believe it. "You did know what you were talking about, didn't you?"

I told her, "You better hurry," as she rolled me down the hallway, and I laughed. "How long do I have?" she asked.

"I'll give you about four good contractions. They are lasting a minute and are a minute apart. It will be about seven minutes."

"Oh, honey, I better hurry!" She barely got me on the delivery table, and I pushed one time as the doctor walked through the door, and our third miracle baby, Miss Lori Dawn, was born. The nurse started scolding me immediately. She said, "You told me I had seven minutes, but you didn't give me but four, and I wasn't ready yet!"

Some doctors do an episiotomy as a routine precaution. We didn't want one and had prayed and had been speaking to my body to stretch. I didn't even have to say anything about it to the doctor. Everything went so fast in the delivery room that he didn't have time to do an episiotomy even if he had planned to.

When the doctor had asked me, several weeks earlier, about an anesthetic, I told him, "I had my last baby without anesthetic, and I don't want to have an anesthetic this time. I did real well and everything went great." I carefully explained that I had two other children and a miscarriage, so I really did know what I was doing. He readily agreed to do whatever I wanted.

He asked, "Do you mind if I have it there, so if you want it, you can ask for it?"

"Sure, that's fine with me," I told him. That didn't offend me at all or hurt my faith. I knew I wouldn't need it and wouldn't ask for it, but if it made him feel better to have it there, it didn't bother me.

The man who was going to administer the anesthetic was sitting right by my head, but he didn't give me any. After it was all over, he just sat there for a minute, even after the doctor left, and talked with me. He said, "In all my career I've never seen anybody have a baby the way you just did. I wish every woman could have her baby like that." Then he got up and started out, turned around at the door and said, "I want you to know you were great!" Then he left. I still laugh when I think about it!

It was amazing to the doctors and nurses. I didn't have to go in there and tell them what all God was going to do. I went in there and did it. They saw a difference and wanted to know why. Then I shared with them and they listened.

Believe Before You Conceive

We had our two boys, and my heart's desire then was to have a little girl. The Bible tells us that God gives us the desires of our heart. (Ps. 37:4.) One night after I put the boys to bed, I told the Lord, "You know my heart's desire: I want a fair-skinned little girl with naturally curly hair, big blue eyes, and a sweet disposition. I want us to have a great friendship just as I had with my mother." I knew I didn't want her to weigh ten pounds, so I said I would like for her to weigh between eight and eight and one-half pounds.

Our third baby was Miss Lori Dawn, eight pounds, four ounces (which is exactly between eight and eight and one-half pounds) with beautiful blond curly hair and big blue eyes. God hears and answers prayer.

Many people after they find out they are going to have a baby decide to start confessing for a particular sex. They get all carried away. "We're painting this room blue because we're confessing this baby is a boy. It would damage our faith if we painted it yellow." It's too late then. If you didn't pray and believe God before that baby was conceived, that's too bad. It's too late. Confessing that your baby is a boy won't change anything after conception. That's like walking over to one of your other children and laying your hands on them and saying, "I confess with my mouth and believe in my heart you're really not a boy; you're a girl." It's the same thing. Just because you don't know what sex it is doesn't mean it's not already determined, because it is and you can't change it with confession. That baby is just as much all girl or just as much all boy at conception as it is at birth. It won't change. You'll know if your faith worked or not when the baby gets here.

Let's be real, folks, not flaky.

5

Can I Be a Joyful Mother of Children?

Something wonderful happened to me when each of my last three babies was born that I didn't understand for several years. As they were born, joy came from way down deep inside of me, and I laughed — out loud. I loved giving birth every time, but it was extra special with the last three babies. The doctors and nurses always commented about the way it was so easy and that they had never seen anyone ever have a baby like that. I didn't understand myself where that thrill and joy came from, but I knew it was very special.

One day as I was sharing this testimony at a luncheon, the Lord spoke through someone who was there and showed me just how it fit together. "That laughter that came from way down inside of you was the joy and the thrill of bringing forth new life. That's the same joy and the same thrill that I feel and all heaven feels when I have a new one born into the kingdom of heaven." I can see that for too long Satan has robbed women of that joy of bringing forth life.

Satan Has a Special Hatred for Women

Satan has a special hatred for women because of the curse God placed on the devil in the Garden.

And the Lord God said unto the serpent, Because thou hast done this, thou art cursed above all cattle, and above every beast of the field; upon thy belly shalt thou go, and dust shalt thou eat all the days of thy life:

> **And I will put enmity between thee and the woman,**
> **and between thy seed and her seed; it shall bruise thy**
> **head, and thou shalt bruise his heel.**
>
> **Genesis 3:14,15**

He has known for all these years that the seed of a woman was going to get him, but he didn't know who the Savior was. He was scared when Moses was born, because he thought it was going to be Moses. In fact, he was scared whenever a prophet was born. He thought, *This is it! This is the one who is going to get me!*

Finally, praise God, Jesus was born, and through His life, death, and resurrection, He totally defeated Satan.

One of the greatest blessings about the whole process of childbirth was that feeling of joy. I had never, ever felt a thrill anything like it. It is a thrill that I feel God has especially given to women — that thrill of bringing forth life.

In fact, to me, there is something so special about even being pregnant. I always enjoyed pregnancy (especially after I realized I could run off sickness). Even before anyone could tell by looking at me that I was pregnant, the baby was such a reality to me; I was conscious of it being there inside of me almost continuously. I felt like I knew a secret — even when everyone else could see I was pregnant. I sometimes felt like I went around with a smile on my face like "the cat that ate the canary." I felt so special. Terry says pregnant women are so pretty, and I think it's the glow of giving life. There is nothing that compares with it except seeing someone born again.

Deal With Fear

Every time something bad comes along, Terry and I always want to know first of all: Where did it come from? Whose fault is it? Why would a woman who is expecting a baby be afraid? Where does this fear come from? Who told her it had to be a bad experience?

This fear is preconceived and is based on what mamma, grandma, television, movies and books have portrayed. In most movies when we see the woman having a baby, she either dies or is in such tormenting pain that she wishes she could die. People share their experiences, and it is rare that the report is good. Usually it is just one horror story after another about how bad it was for them and that it won't be any better for you. That's natural for people to do. They believe it and confess it, and they have their confession working against them. For the world that's fairly accurate, but we're not of the world. The Bible says we are in this world but not of this world. (John 17:14.)

Many of the doctors and nurses I have talked to say the worst enemy of a pregnant woman in labor is fear.

You'll find that fear is your number one enemy no matter what you're doing. The opposite of fear is faith. When you're believing God for your health, for your finances, for your family or for anything else, fear is your number one enemy.

But we know what to do with fear. Say out loud, "I rebuke you fear in the name of Jesus. God has not given me a spirit of fear, but of power, and of love, and of a sound mind. I have God's perfect love and that perfect love casts out fear." (2 Tim. 1:7; 1 John 4:18.) You rebuke fear, and fear leaves. But that's a continuous thing. Fear doesn't just leave and stay gone forever. It will come around again when you least expect it. So you need to learn to recognize the first symptom of fear, deal with it, get rid of it and go on.

And you can do it! I did it! When the contractions came, and I would start tightening up and getting scared, I'd talk to my body, very quietly — nobody ever heard me or knew what I was doing — but it was loud enough for me, God and the devil to hear. Recognize fear and command it to leave in Jesus' name, and it has to go. **Submit yourselves therefore to God. Resist the devil, and he will flee from you** (James 4:7).

None Shall Be Barren

The Lord said in Psalm 113:9: **He maketh the barren woman to keep house, and to be a joyful mother of children.**

We have had many couples come to us and tell us that either because they could not conceive or because of multiple miscarriages, "We can't have children."

We have been able to share good news with them: God says you can have children.

Lo, children are an heritage of the Lord: and the fruit of the womb is his reward.

As arrows are in the hand of a mighty man; so are children of the youth.

Happy is the man that hath his quiver full of them: they shall not be ashamed, but they shall speak with the enemies in the gate.

Psalm 127:3-5

Thy wife shall be as a fruitful vine by the sides of thine house: thy children like olive plants round about thy table.

Psalm 128:3

And he will love thee, and bless thee, and multiply thee: he will also bless the fruit of thy womb...

Thou shalt be blessed above all people: there shall not be male or female barren among you.

Deuteronomy 7:13,14

There shall nothing cast their young, nor be barren, in thy land: the number of thy days I will fulfil.

Exodus 23:26

And if you are a tither, you also have Malachi 3:10,11:

Bring ye all the tithes into the storehouse, that there may be meat in mine house, and prove me now herewith, saith the Lord of hosts, if I will not open you the windows of heaven, and pour you out a blessing, that there shall not be room enough to receive it.

And I will rebuke the devourer for your sakes, and he shall not destroy the fruits of your ground; neither shall your vine cast her fruit before the time in the field, saith the Lord of hosts.

"Casting your fruit before its time" refers, of course, to a miscarriage.

There was a young couple who had already had about four miscarriages when we met them. We had known some of their relatives for a long time, and although we had not met them, we had heard about them. Their family had told us, "It's so sad. It's really a shame. They just can't seem to have a baby. She gets pregnant, but then she miscarries every time." You can tell they had the power of agreement working against them.

When we met those kids, we started sharing the Word with them. We told them they could stand on God's Word, and God would honor His Word and be faithful to them. Well, the girl conceived again.

One night she started bleeding, and they called Terry. He went to their house, shared with them, encouraged them, and prayed with them. She didn't miscarry. In fact, God is so neat, not only did she not miscarry, she had identical twins! That's God! That's the way He operates! Give Him half a chance and He will bless you abundantly — more than you could ask or even think. (Eph. 3:20.)

The world tells you all you can't do, never have been able to and never will. But God's provision is: when you are established in His Word, you can do anything. You can change your life totally. You can change anything to line up with what God's Word says.

We had another friend, Edith Reese, who, although she had one baby, had been unable to have another one. She had six miscarriages. Friends, relatives, everyone around her said, "I don't know how she had that one, but she'll never have another one. She just can't carry it."

The doctors told Edith that she was not developed inside: she was like a twelve-year-old girl. Her cervix and uterus were not normal or healthy. The doctors suggested sewing up her cervix to keep the fetus from aborting if she did get pregnant. The doctors and many others said if she became pregnant she would have to stay flat in bed for the full nine months.

Edith and her husband, Gene, asked us to pray for them to have a baby. Terry asked Edith if she could believe for a baby. "I don't think so," she told him.

"Can you believe in our prayers and faith," he asked her, "that if we pray you'll have a baby?"

"I don't know," she answered.

"Okay, can you agree with us that the Bible is the Word of God and that God's Word is truth?"

"Yes, I can do that," she said.

"Can you agree with me when I pray and I say that you will conceive and you'll not lose this baby, because you are redeemed from the curse?" he asked.

"Well, I don't know. I've had so many miscarriages," she answered.

Terry said, "Let's go back to the Bible. Can you agree with what God says?"

"Yes, I can agree with God."

"That's all I want you to do. I want you to say, `I agree with what God says: that I'll conceive and I'll not lose my baby. I'll not cast my fruit before its time. I will have a healthy, whole baby because I am redeemed from the curse, according to Galatians 3:13, and I will have this baby.'"

"I can do that," she said.

We prayed for her, and she started saying what God said on this. Of course she conceived and called us with the good news.

They went on a trip by car — from Texas to California and back to Texas (over three thousand miles) — when she was only two months along. While they were gone, she started bleeding. They called us and we prayed. She just kept saying what God said. She said, "No, I won't lose this baby. I agree with what God says. Christ has redeemed me from the curse of the law. I'll not cast my fruit before its time."

She had that baby, a beautiful little girl. The doctors remarked that the membrane of the sac that contains the baby was so thick they had to break it for her to deliver. God had put His own supernatural safeguard in place for that baby! But do you know what? People would have talked her out of having that baby if she had listened to them. You have to totally separate your thinking from the old ways and completely renew your mind. (Rom. 12:2.)

I'm not telling you that I've never had a negative thought. I've had the same dumb thoughts that most pregnant women have had. It's the same devil that comes and tells me all those stupid things. But I've learned to recognize him more quickly now so I don't listen nearly as long as I used to.

Almost two years to the day after Lori was born, our fourth child, Miss Cristy Denise, arrived. Now, according to the doctor, she was one week overdue. In fact, he had told me if I didn't have her before my next appointment with him — which was on Thursday — he would induce labor. By that Wednesday I had begun to have a bloody show and knew the time was near.

As my mother and I put supper on the table that evening, I decided not to eat — I didn't feel like there was room for food anyway, the baby seemed so big. By 8:00 that night I began having regular contractions, about five minutes apart. (I had asked the Lord to let me know when to go to the hospital so I wouldn't be rushed. I wanted to have time to check in, fill out the papers, and still have time to feel I was together and in control of things.)

At 9:00 p.m. we decided we should go to the hospital so I could be checked. My contractions were regular and getting stronger...until we got there. Then I didn't have another contraction for almost twenty minutes. The nurses checked me and said, "You're only dilated three centimeters and your labor is irregular. You won't have this baby tonight. Why don't you just go on home?" (I had been dilated three centimeters for a month.)

I said, "Please let me stay a little while." I told them that I really did know what I was doing, that I had babies so fast and so easily that there wouldn't be time for me to go home and get back. Within the time it took me to convince them to let me stay, the contractions started again, this time much harder and five minutes apart.

During the short labor, I was doing so well I became over-confident. The contractions were very hard on the monitor and there was no pain. Having wondered about the focal point, panting and breathing that women are taught in natural childbirth classes, I decided to try it. Boy, was that a mistake! I don't know what I was thinking, but the minute I began to pant and breathe it was as though my trust and confidence moved to the natural and was no longer in God and His Word. And natural ability isn't enough. I had about three contractions that really hurt before I realized what I had done and got back on God's Word, in authority and in control and without pain!

At 10:45 p.m. the nurse yelled for the doctor to hurry and get in the delivery room. As he rushed in, putting on his gloves, she was holding Cristy's head in me with a towel to prevent her from coming out before the doctor was ready.

What a thrill to experience the joy of giving birth again! I've always said Cristy was our good measure, pressed down, shaken together and running over abundant blessing. She has always been the icing on the cake for us.

The next morning a nurse came in my room with my chart in her hand. She said, "I was getting everyone ready for their sitz bath, and I saw you weren't scheduled for one. I had to come in here and see with my own eyes the lady who had a nine-pound, five-ounce baby and doesn't have any stitches. That must be a miracle." She didn't know how much of a miracle it really was.

There comes a time when you have to stand on the Word of God and say, "No, I reject the defeat and the disappointments of the past. I'm not receiving that anymore. I'm going to stand on God's Word and have God's best."

You'll have to do whatever it takes to overcome in your circumstance, like we did in our situation. When the doctors said I could never have a baby, I couldn't accept that. It was the overwhelming desire of my heart to have children. I couldn't stand not having a family. So we stood on the Word and grew in the Word, and the Word produced for us four children — two boys and two girls. As far as I'm concerned, we have a perfect family. You should have a perfect family too. Four may not be the perfect number for you, but however many you want, you can have them by using the Word of God. The Word will produce for you just as it did for us.

We have received many testimonies from women with whom we have prayed and shared the Word. They are now what the Bible says they would be — "a joyful mother of children."

6
Face the Issue

Many times we get concerned with things that are petty, and we actually miss the real issue. There is now a "great debate" going on over where Christian women should have their babies and who should deliver them. Opinions include: have the baby at home, at a birthing center, or at a hospital; delivery should be done by the husband, a midwife or a doctor. Then there are numerous combinations of the above. Folks, that's not even the issue. God doesn't care where you have your baby. It makes absolutely no difference to Him. The decision is yours. It's a matter of personal preference.

"But can you go to the hospital and really be in faith and believing God?" some have asked.

You need to be believing God wherever you plan to have that baby. The issue is not whether to go to the hospital, the issue is to end up with a healthy mother and a healthy baby. Isn't that simple? Just do what you have to, to get that result.

One lady came to me quite upset because I went to the doctor and had my babies in a hospital. That isn't the point. The point is either to have fear and pain and do the best you can, or to believe God to have it supernaturally without fear and pain, without problems, without complications. You can do either, either place. And God doesn't care, but He did make a way for you.

There are many people, even preachers, who are saying, "You must have your baby at home." I don't want to get into that controversy. Just let me tell you, in general, don't ever let a preacher or anyone else, for that matter, make that decision for you. It is none of their business where you have your baby. You have to be responsible for your own decision.

Some women have said, "God told me to have my baby at home." Basically, God doesn't care where you have your baby. Now there may be a rare situation in which, because the woman was believing God in another area of her health, certain medical procedures would automatically be initiated but actually would not be needed because of God's intervention. In such a case the woman might feel she could use her faith more effectively at home and not have to submit to unnecessary procedures. God could move in an area like that and give her confidence that that's exactly what she was supposed to do — stay home and have her baby. But like I said, that would be a rare instance.

We have had to deal with so many people who have stayed home and made messes that it's almost unbelievable. They stay home saying they are believing God, but when you get down to it, they couldn't believe God for the finances to pay the hospital. If you can't believe for the money to pay a hospital bill, then you can't believe God and be responsible for a human life.

Women have been having babies for centuries. You can have your baby at the hospital, at home, in a barn, in the field, anywhere you want to have it as far as God is concerned. It is merely a matter of personal preference.

I will say this, if you're going to have it at home, then you better know what you're doing, and you better have someone there who is qualified because I'm tired of God getting a black eye over this. People say God told them to have their baby at home, and then the baby dies, or the mother almost dies, and God gets the blame. And one more time Christians look like flakes.

A pastor, who is a close friend of ours, called Terry one day at 4:00 a.m. as Terry was preparing to leave for Mexico. The pastor said, "Terry, would you please call this couple from my church? The woman says that God told her to have her baby at home. Her water broke twenty-four hours ago, and she's still not in labor; nothing is happening. She won't go to the doctor or the hospital. Would you call her and talk to her?"

"Do I know them?"

"No, but they know you. I think they will listen to you."

So Terry called, and the husband answered. After Terry identified himself, he asked to talk to the wife. Her husband said she would not come to the phone. Finally Terry said, "Listen, God didn't tell her to have her baby at home. If He had, it would be working. You better pack her up and take her to the hospital. Now let me talk to your wife!"

"Sister, I want you to go to the hospital, and let them see about you," Terry told her.

"No," she said, "I'm not going to do it. God told me not to go to the hospital."

"God did not tell you that. Let me ask you a question? Have you had a baby before?"

"No."

"If you'd had a baby before, then I would tell you it's none of my business because you know what you're doing. Once a woman has had a baby, she knows what's going on. But you don't know what you're doing. Have you even been to the doctor to be examined?"

Again the answer was no.

Terry continued, "I feel in my spirit that you're too small to even have that baby. I don't know what you look like; I just have that in my spirit. If you've never been to the doctor to be examined, you may be in for trouble. Do you know how dangerous this could be?"

"No," she answered.

Terry told her, "I want you to go to the hospital now!"

"No, I'm not going. I'm standing in faith," she said. "But I am a little frustrated because my mom had all her babies breech, and I think my baby might be breech."

"You're not standing in faith! Frustration is not faith. And after twenty-four hours, you're tired and worn out. I'm going to tell you something very plain. I'm not trying to damage your faith, but I'd rather damage your faith than have you kill your baby. Your faith is repairable, but your baby is not replaceable. You are not in faith. Faith works, and if it's not working, there is something wrong. Go to the hospital now."

She refused.

"All I can do for you is pray." Terry prayed, "Father, I believe You to give them the mind of Christ and the wisdom of God." He spoke again to the husband and told him, "I don't care what you have to do, get her to the hospital now." He hung up and left for Mexico for a crusade.

When he returned from Mexico, he immediately called that pastor for a report on the lady. The pastor said, "Her husband grabbed her up, put her in the car and drove to the hospital. The doctor examined her and said that she was too small — there was no way she could deliver that baby. They took the baby by Caesarean section; it weighed nine pounds. It could have killed her and the baby too. She's mad at you and her husband because the doctor told her she can never deliver a baby normally now since she has had a Caesarean section."

She stayed mad for several weeks.

The next time we went to that city, she came up and hugged Terry and me. She was crying and said, "I'm so glad you made me go. I wouldn't have my baby. Now I'm using my faith to believe my hip bones will spread so I can deliver my next one normally." You see, she didn't even know what to believe for; now she does.

The best time to use your faith for having babies is before you ever get pregnant.

Know Your Faith Level

I have a tape out on supernatural childbirth. Many people get hold of it and listen to it over and over and over until it becomes so real to them that it works for them. Any woman who is average, normal, can pick up that tape, find out what the Word of God says and have a baby without pain, without anesthetic, without problems, stitches, or nausea. But that's an average situation. There is nothing wrong with her; everything is normal; she's average. Then having a baby is not a problem. Women have been doing it for thousands of years — at home, in hospitals, in a manger (like Mary), anywhere. God doesn't care.

But see, that woman wasn't average. She had to believe God for a creative miracle to get to be average and she didn't even know it. She thought that she was just believing God to have a baby.

But if a woman is below average, then she needs to build her faith to get to average, normal. And she needs to start believing for supernatural childbirth before she conceives.

I was below average. The first time I was pregnant and miscarried, Terry told me, "It will never happen again. I'll get in the Bible, and it will never happen again." We were believing God for a miracle to get to average. We had three years before Lynn was born. In those three years we used the name of Jesus, we used our faith — what little we knew — and we used the Bible.

When I conceived Lynn, we were away from everyone who knew us, and I didn't tell the army doctors any of the bad reports other doctors had given me. I had an uncomplicated pregnancy, but when the army doctors ran tests, they said I was a gestation diabetic. I was still below average. We prayed and believed God. And although the doctors planned to induce labor because they were afraid the baby was too big, God intervened and I went into labor before time, and we got what we believed for — a fast, uncomplicated delivery.

We continued to study the Word and build our faith and confidence in God in the area of childbearing. The next time I conceived, God did a miracle and brought me up to average. The next three children were "supernatural" — just as God always intended.

We all need to realize where our faith level is. You may have all the faith in the world but if you're below average, you're going to have to use all that faith to get to average.

People are on different levels of physical ability. Now, if there were two women who were both average, and only one of them used her faith, she would excel and the other one wouldn't. But if there's a woman who is below normal, then she needs the Word to get her up to normal, average.

There are some people — Christians and sinners — who are normal. That was Terry's case. There wasn't anything wrong with him; there still isn't; there never will be. And he took the Word of God and started building on that, and he built that into me and into the kids. We're building on that all the time. It's our foundation.

But some people have to have a miracle to get to average. Some people have things wrong with them. Instead of being average and going up, they are below average and to get to average, they need a miracle.

Be encouraged; stay with it. God will meet you where you are and bring you where you need to be.

7

Conclusion

People often fight for the right to suffer. I'm not trying to push off any doctrine on anybody. I'm just saying what the Word says. The Word says you can do things God's way. You can do things other ways as well. You can be sick, and God will still love you. You can be poor, and God will still love you. You can be barren, and God will still love you. You can live in pain, and God will still love you. But God says there is a better way. Jesus has paid for salvation, healing, prosperity, deliverance and blessing.

God is so practical. God is so real. He wants you to do what you can do, what you can handle. He wants to bless you. He wants to meet your needs. He wants you to walk in health and prosperity and all the blessings that He has given you through Jesus. He'll do anything to meet you where you are if you put your confidence in Him and His Word. God will always be there to back up His Word.

I want to emphasize: God wants to bless you. Never let the devil condemn you or push you into doing something just because someone else did it. Remember, the issue is to have a healthy mother and a healthy baby. Study the Bible and decide for yourself where you will draw the line. God loves you just the way you are, and wherever you are is where He'll meet you.

If this book has helped you in any way, we'd love to hear from you. Send us your testimony, and if that testimony includes the birth of a precious little baby, we'd love for you to send us pictures. Terry and I are privileged to have the opportunity to share the goodness of God with you. If you need prayer, encouragement or just want to share with someone, please write to us. We will pray for you and be in agreement with you for God's very best.

8
Testimonies

We've included a few testimonies we've received as a result of the tape we've had out called "Supernatural Childbirth." Rejoice, as we have, with these people; be encouraged by their testimonies, and know for a certainty that what God has done for others He will do for you. God is no respecter of persons. Abide in the Word of God and let His Word abide in you and you can ask what you will and it will be done for you. (Acts 10:34, John 15:7.)

Dear Jackie . . .

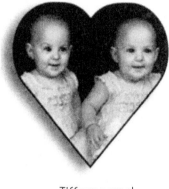

Tiffany and
Andrea Davis

Soon after Jerry and I decided to start a family, we were excited to know that we were expecting a baby. We were very disappointed when I miscarried a few weeks later. Over the course of the next two years I had three more miscarriages – none of the pregnancies lasted longer than six to eight weeks.

As this seemingly hopeless pattern developed, we realized that we had a real problem. Jerry and I both went through a series of tests, saw several doctors and tried medications to determine if something could be corrected physically. Nothing we did gave us any answer to why this was happening.

We knew if we were going to have children God would have to give them to us, but we didn't know how to effectively stand on the Word for our miracle.

About the time of my fourth miscarriage is when you and Terry learned of our problem and began sharing with us principles in the Word we could use to build our faith so that we could receive from God. Jackie, you shared Scripture with me which gave specific answers that I needed. I quoted these often.

With this new knowledge, the fifth pregnancy was quite different. I carried this one past the critical eight-week period with no problem. I had never felt better than during those months of that pregnancy.

In the sixth month I began showing the familiar signs of miscarriage. Just days earlier, I had seen my doctor during one of my routine visits. He told me if I should deliver from that time on we had a "good chance of saving the baby." Because of my medical history, he was monitoring me very closely. I knew he meant what he said as encouragement, but I refused to settle for less than seeing this pregnancy through to full term. Satan was trying to use the doctor's words, along with my physical symptoms, to make me give up, deliver early and risk losing the baby.

Initially, fear came, but I quickly overcame it with the Word that I had been confessing and living in the previous months. Soon all the symptoms disappeared. Praise God for the knowledge I had gained with your help!

Early in the seventh month, the same doctor sent me for an ultrasound because he thought he heard two heartbeats. That ultrasound revealed I was carrying twins. What a reward this news was after winning the battle we had faced just a few weeks earlier.

Jackie, you had also shared with me how you learned that we do not have to go through pain during childbirth. I wanted all God had for me, so I claimed the promises in the Word pertaining to that too. If God could help me carry this pregnancy, He could take away the pain of delivery. When I did go into labor, it was hard to know when it was actually time to go to the hospital because I had no pain.

On March 6, 1977 I gave birth to beautiful, perfectly healthy twin daughters: Tiffany Danielle, three pounds, thirteen ounces and Andrea Gabrielle, four pounds, fourteen ounces. It was as though God was making up for lost time by giving us twins. We are so thankful to God for giving us our miracle in a way much greater than anything we could have every imagined.

Melinda Davis
Conroe, Texas

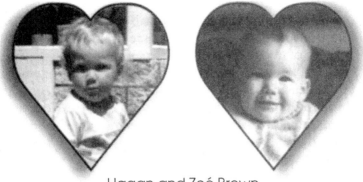

Hagan and Zoé Brown

G ordon and I have three children, two I had supernaturally according to the Word of God.

Our first baby was born with a congenital deformity of the lower leg and later had to have an amputation. He now wears an artificial limb. Along with that, the whole birth process of labor was full of complications and fear.

Doctors began to tell us they were not sure if this could happen to us again. I then had two miscarriages. All this increased the fear I had.

Then someone gave me your tape, "Supernatural Childbirth." Even though I had been a Christian all this time, I didn't know it didn't have to be this way. After the second miscarriage, doctors told me I was not to conceive for at least six months. So I took your tape and listened to it every day for the next six months. I was determined to build my faith to the place where I knew I could have a baby.

At the end of that six months, Terry was in New Zealand, so we had him pray and agree with us. Nine months later I held my completely healthy baby, who was born in four hours, without complications.

With our third baby, again I had no trouble conceiving. She was born very quickly – just over an hour, with no pain, stitches or complications.

I knew this was the way God intended for women to have babies. Gordon and I are so thankful to God for His Word.

Julie Brown
New Plymouth, New Zealand

This is a second generation supernatural childbirth testimony. Edith believed the Word of God and reaped the reward by giving birth to Leanna.

(See Chapter 5.)

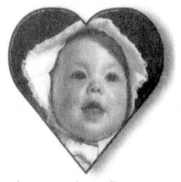

Leanna Jean Reese

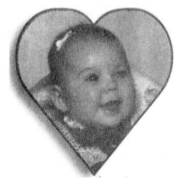

Brittini Jordan Reese

My daughter, Leanna, at age fifteen years became pregnant. She was a sophomore in high school and continued attending school (one that used paces – independent study), doing so well she started her junior year work. She was ninety-six pounds and five feet three inches tall when she got pregnant.

Beginning in her third month, she started listening to your tape on supernatural childbirth almost every night. She got out her Bible and looked up all the Scriptures and typed them out. She confessed she would have an easy

71

delivery and that every part of the baby would be perfect and complete. There would be no complications during the pregnancy or afterward.

The last two weeks of May she had contractions but no pain. She was dilated to 4 cm. for a little over one week. At her doctor's appointment, May 30, he decided to put her in the hospital June 2. At 7:30 a.m. on that Saturday she entered the hospital – she still didn't even know she was in labor. Her baby girl, Brittini Jordan, six pounds five and one-half ounces, was born at 10:36 a.m. The nurses and doctor said she did great! They were surprised how quickly she had the baby, especially because it was her first – she was so young and so small. She had some stitches from the baby being so big, but other than being tired, she was fine.

Leanna, with the help and support of her husband, is a joyful mother and a high school graduate!

The same Word of God that brought our daughter Leanna into the world gave us our precious granddaughter, Brittini.

Edith Reese
New Mexico

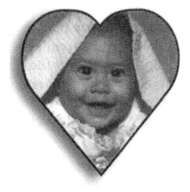

Ashley Sepulveda

In my freshman year at high school, in 1973, I watched a film in a P.E. class on natural childbirth. I was so negatively affected by that film and the awful pain that woman was displaying, that

I didn't think I'd ever have a baby of my own. I thought I could not handle the pain and would just as well adopt.

Although I realize it's pretty common for a young girl to feel the way I did, I didn't seem to get rid of that way of thinking, even after I was born again in 1978 or after I was married in 1982.

I tried to convince my husband that adoption was the best. I think he accepted that when we were first married because he wasn't thinking of children at that time – but I knew at the back of his mind he wanted to have our own.

Two years into our marriage I was given your tape, "Supernatural Childbirth." I had never heard that term before or that painless delivery was possible, but I was very interested in knowing more about it. I listened and listened and listened to it. By the latter part of 1984, being confident that God was no respecter of people, your words of faith rang out in my heart and mind. "If we're redeemed from the curse of the law, then we are. If we are, we are!" That phrase of faith-filled words brought deliverance to me. I believed that it was true for me (and for every believer, as well).

I shared my faith – and the tape – with my husband, Art. He agreed that God was able and willing to watch over His Word and perform it in our lives. Pain is under the curse, and I was set free from pain and the fear of it, as well.

I conceived in April 1985 and in my sixth week experienced symptoms of a miscarriage. But I stood on my covenant rights and told my body that it would not drop its fruit before the time (because I was and am a tither). I spoke John 10:10 and let it be my dividing line: God placed this baby in my womb to be filled with His life and His life more abundantly. I continued listening to your tape and practically quoting your words of life together with you as you spoke. The week after all the symptoms said I was going to lose my baby I went to my doctor, and he said my blood count was right on track and that everything was fine.

About eight months later at 2:00 a.m. I went to the hospital with contractions. They felt like a lot of pressure on my vagina and all around by abdomen, but there was no pain. My legs began to shake a bit while I was in labor. When I asked the nurses why, they said, "You're trying to be a wonder-woman and probably need a pain killer. I said, "No, I don't have any pain, but I just can't seem to make my legs stop shaking."

After about twelve hours of a lot of pressure on and off lasting about one to two minutes, every three to four minutes for twelve hours, Ashley was born. No pain! In fact, I kept pushing even after Ashley was already out because I didn't feel her come out of me.

I have shared this tape with every pregnant woman who wanted it. I even gave one to a co-worker while I was working for an airline in Reservations. She became born again while listening to it. She also had a vaginal birth when her doctor said she was too small (and because she had a Cesarean section with her first child). After receiving your tape about two weeks into her seventh month, she called me crying and said, "My bones are moving. I spoke to my body like Jackie said, and I know God is making the adjustments so that I can have this baby naturally...I mean supernaturally." And she did!

Thank you, Jackie, for being willing to share yourself and your testimony with so many of us who have been mightily blessed.

Kuna Sepulveda
Honolulu, Hawaii

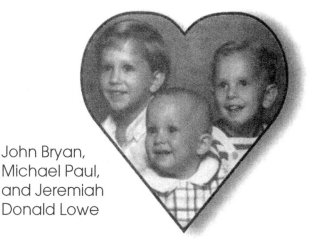

John Bryan,
Michael Paul,
and Jeremiah
Donald Lowe

R ight after my husband and I were born again and
Spirit filled, we heard your testimony about how
you were told by doctors that you couldn't have
children, but because of believing God and His Word,
you now had four healthy children. My husband and I
decided to believe God to conceive.

It had been three and one-half years since we lost our
first child, just a few short weeks away from my due date.
We were told by our doctor that I would probably never
carry a child full term. My husband, at that point a
sophomore in college playing college football, decided to
throw himself into his football career and started taking
steroids, which added to the complications of getting
pregnant and having a baby.

I hadn't conceived yet in over three and one-half years,
even though we hadn't used any birth control; but because
of hearing your testimony on how to believe God for a
miracle, we now had faith sparked in us. Our pastors
prayed for us for healing, and in three months I conceived.

Complications with the pregnancy set in right away, but

we knew it was God's will for us to have a baby, so we just kept believing.

We were visiting with you when I was seven months pregnant, and we shared that we were going through natural childbirth classes to prepare for this baby. I will never forget Terry's response, "Why have natural childbirth when you can have supernatural childbirth?" He then went on to share about how to have a supernatural delivery by the Word.

When we went home, I listened over and over again to the tape you gave us of your testimony. I made a prayer confession from the tape to speak the Word to my body and the baby even though we were still getting negative reports about the baby each time we went to the doctor. I can't say that my first delivery was pain free, but it was a miracle!

Contrary to what the doctor expected, I gave birth to a healthy seven-pound and fourteen-ounce baby boy, John Bryan Lowe III.

When I conceived again, my faith was built up; I was ready to trust God for a pain-free delivery. I had trouble with my water breaking with John Bryan, so that was one specific thing that I believed God for the next time. I was expecting this one to be quick.

When the time came, my water broke at home, and I went into labor. We set out for the hospital, which was a twenty-minute drive. Fifteen minutes after we got there, Jeremiah Donald Lowe was born. When we got to the hospital and they examined me, I was so surprised that I was in the last transition of labor. I felt the baby coming, and when I stood up, he crowned. In a few minutes the nurses had me in the bed.

I was lying there so elated by the fact that I wasn't in pain that the doctor had to get my attention and remind me to push. So I pushed two times and Jeremiah was here! The doctors and nurses were so amazed at the ease of my delivery, they all gave me a standing ovation after the delivery. I felt so overwhelmed about being free from pain. I just kept thinking, Well of course this is how God would want it to be because it was so wonderful!

The next baby came two and one-half years later, and the devil really tried to complicate this one. I was in labor without pain, and I knew it was time to go to the hospital. When they examined me, the doctors told us the baby was coming double foot breach. They wanted to do an emergency C-Section right away.

We asked the doctors for a few minutes of privacy to pray. They were exasperated and concerned, but they conceded to leave us alone. We then did what you and Terry taught us to do, we laid hands on my stomach and prayed over the baby. We commanded the baby to move and get in the right position in the name of Jesus. We spoke to my body. We did everything we could think of.

The doctors came back in and re-examined me and insisted on a C-Section. Michael Paul Lowe was born by way of a C-Section, a healthy, normal six-pound and three-ounce beautiful baby boy. The following day the doctor came to my room. He told us that when they made the incision, they found the baby head first. We were informed that had the doctors waited we could have had a natural vaginal delivery, which they assured us was impossible, due to the baby's original footing breach position. We saw that as a real victory!

I truly appreciate you and Terry sharing with us about trusting in God's Word. It is true, and it works in my life!

Debbie Lowe
Warsaw, Indiana

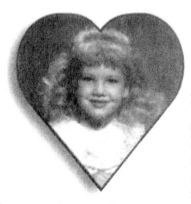

Jessica Burke

It was a wonderful day when I heard you share your principles for raising a successful family. You represented to me a seasoned woman of God who had pursued His will and ministry but without sacrificing your children's well being.

Dennis and I had been happily married for ten years. We were in a traveling ministry, and I considered us quite fulfilled. We agreed in all areas except one – children. I felt that since we traveled full time it was best not to have any children, while Dennis wanted a family. But he knew my answers would have to come from God. He only prayed that God would change me.

It wasn't that I disliked children, but I had strong convictions about being a good parent. Even though Dennis and I agreed on how children should be raised, that didn't seem to fit into our lifestyle. We felt God wouldn't want me to stay home through long separations from Dennis, nor would He want us to leave our children to be raised by someone else. My solution was simply not to have children.

It seems impossible now to realize how I was limiting God. It never occurred to me that there was another way. It never dawned on me that Jesus is the Way, and He could easily show me how to work it out.

In 1979 we attended the International Convention of Faith Ministries conference in Fort Worth, Texas. One afternoon at a ladies' meeting, a panel of trustees' wives opened the floor for questions. When a woman asked about children, the entire panel directed the question to you, Jackie.

You spoke as though you knew my thoughts and misgivings. Your practical answers brought me such freedom that I was forever changed. Your words showed me that children did not need to suffer because of our type of ministry and travel. Instead, they could be a vital part of all we did and have the added advantage of world travel.

I spent the next few years observing your whole family, just to see how it worked for you. Anyone who spends time with you, especially enjoys being around your children. As a result of the wisdom you shared, today Dennis and I have a beautiful and well-adjusted daughter who travels with us around the world.

Thank you, Jackie, for pointing me to the Way-maker.

Vikki Burke
Arlington, Texas

listened to your tape "Supernatural Childbirth" for several years before our daughter Ruthi was conceived. I found the principles you teach to be practical and helpful in all areas of my life, enabling me to prepare for a wonderful pregnancy and delivery. I

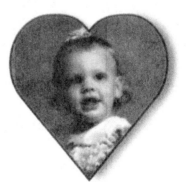

Ruthi McNerlin

experienced no morning sickness during my pregnancy and, despite the doctors' warnings of a long, uncomfortable first delivery, I was only in labor for five hours and twenty-five minutes.

My water broke and the doctor induced contractions several hours later. They weren't overbearing, but tiring, so I opted for an epidural. The nurses told me I wasn't dilating very quickly and that I would be there for a while. George and I just smiled, and when they left the room, we prayed. I dilated almost immediately – much to their surprise. Through the main part of my labor I watched a football game and laughed and talked with my family! (My mom said I would have had more than one brother if she had had deliveries like mine!)

Again, the nurses were surprised when I was ready to deliver much sooner than they expected. However, they advised me it could still take time. Within twenty minutes I was holding our baby! My doctor really chuckled when only minutes after Ruthi's birth I said, "If that's all there is to it, I'll have twelve!"

With much prayer and use of the knowledge I gained from you and from my doctor, God blessed us with a wonderful delivery. I have recommended the tape "Supernatural Childbirth" to many women and am thrilled to finally see it in print. I believe women everywhere will be encouraged by the wisdom you share.

Nita McNerlin
Katy, Texas

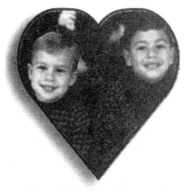

Dominic Joseph and
Jonathan Michael Russo

My heart is filled with joy and excitement as I begin to share with you my personal testimony on supernatural childbirth. The Lord has blessed me with two beautiful sons, Dominic Joseph and Jonathan Michael; both love the Lord and want all that God has for them.

When I first found out I was pregnant with Dominic in February of 1983, I immediately remembered your tape on supernatural childbirth which had been given to me by a precious sister in the Lord.

The first time I listened to the tape, I knew that I knew that I was to believe God for a supernatural childbirth. My wonderful husband, Dominic Jr., listened to the tape with me and agreed with me for a supernatural childbirth, a God-glorifying delivery and for all of God's promises pertaining to childbirth. It was a blessing to have my husband standing with me on God's Word for a blessed delivery. I had a beautiful pregnancy with Dominic Joseph. I had no morning sickness, no complications whatsoever. I listened to your tape while I put on my makeup, daily, for nine months. When it came time for delivery, I was so full of God's promises for a supernatural, God-glorifying delivery. Your testimony was so encouraging; I just knew God was no respecter of persons, and what God did for you, He would do for me. (Rom. 2:11.)

I had great expectations as I went to the hospital ready to give birth to my first son. I had a beautiful delivery with Dominic – very little pain; I dilated quickly and easily and only had to push twice. After I had given birth to Dominic, I thought, "If I ever get pregnant again, I know now what to expect during labor," and I knew my next childbirth would be totally pain free.

In September of 1985 I found I was pregnant with my second son, Jonathan; he was due April 7, 1986. I was so excited to experience childbirth for the second time. I began listening to your tape again and thanking God for a supernatural childbirth with no pain. Again I had a great nine months carrying Jonathan – no sickness, perfect health. On Saturday, March 22, I went to breakfast with my husband, son and in-laws. We went to the mall and walked around that afternoon. My husband, my son, and I returned home. That evening I told my husband, "I feel like my muscles are getting ready for labor," I went to bed that evening at 8:00 p.m., which is unusual for me.

At 3:00 a.m. the alarm went off, my husband was going to the prison in Muskegon, Michigan for prison ministry. As he was in the shower, I felt in my heart my labor was starting. I had no real pain, but just a bloody show. My mind was telling me "But you're two weeks early." My heart was saying, "It's time."

My husband met the men at the church office who were going to the prison and told them I was in labor and he wouldn't be able to go with them. He prayed with the men from the church to have a fruitful time of ministry as they ministered to the men in prison. As Dominic returned home from the church office he said to me, "This better be it because if it isn't, it's going to look like I didn't want to go to the prison." At that time I knew I was going to have a baby that morning. I showered, called my dear mother over to watch my son. I called our pastor and his wife for prayer, and the church prayed for me as well. There's nothing like a whole church body standing with you! My husband and I arrived at the hospital about 8:45 a.m. Dominic and I had prayed for a specific doctor to deliver my child; he was on call.

As the doctor examined me (he was ready to go off duty at 9:00 a.m.) he said, "I will stay to deliver your baby; it probably won't be until tonight." (I was only dilated to 2 cm.) I had no real consistent contractions, but I knew my body was going to have the baby soon.

When the doctor examined me around 10:00 a.m., I was dilated to 5 cm. Minutes later I had the urge to push, and I told the nurse please to check me again. She said, "There's no way, you were just examined."

I told her, "I know I'm ready." She called a resident to check me, and sure enough I was ready to push. No one could believe how fast I had dilated. I felt this delivery was just like one you described on your tape. I had my second son at 10:20 a.m. with absolutely no pain! God is so good; He loves us so much. My son Jonathan weighed 6 pounds 7 ounces, and he is adorable. I love him very much.

It was such a blessing how the doctor had stayed on for us. The next morning when he came into my room he told me I had done a beautiful job. I was so blessed, filled with joy and happiness. Having a baby is a wonderful experience with the Lord, your husband and those you love around. What a testimony to have a God glorifying delivery. I couldn't believe I had Jonathan two weeks early, but I believe God knew our perfect due date. He was born on Palm Sunday, March 23, 1986.

I can't begin to tell you how many people I have shared supernatural childbirth with. I keep copies of your tape in my briefcase and am constantly giving them out to people. What a wonderful tool for people to listen to, so they can also believe God for a God glorifying delivery. Thank you Jackie for sharing your testimony with us.

Amira Russo
Rochester, Michigan

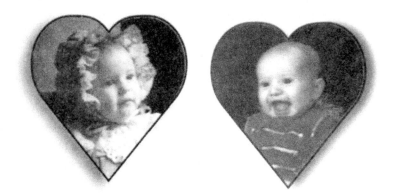

Destiny Rambo and Israel Anthem McGuire

hristians are amazing. When I first heard the tape of "Supernatural Childbirth" I was so excited, I began to tell all my family and friends expecting them to say, "Praise God, isn't this fabulous!" Instead, they looked at me and my swollen belly, raised their eyebrows, rubbed their noses, and generally gave me one of those "Bless your heart, you've gone off the deep end" looks. I should have been used to it by that time.

My husband, Dony, and I had fought the war over our seed for several years. I'd gone through two miscarriages, two corrective surgeries, several humiliating procedures, and finally a grim prognosis: "If you want children, you had better pursue adoption." Now I must tell you, we didn't have a problem with adoption, but we did have a problem in that God had given us several prophetic words about my giving birth. The first week we were married, God had shown me a vision of our son, Israel.

The real breakthrough had occurred when Dony was in prayer one day, and he cried out in his spirit. "God, Your first commandment to mankind was to be fruitful and multiply. Reba and I are Your covenant children, and we expect to be able to keep all Your commandments. We declare the curse of barrenness is broken!"

Six weeks later, I was pregnant! Immediately the skeptics showed up. "Don't get too excited...remember your history of miscarriage." I admit, I wasn't too spiritual at that point. I just wanted to slug them.

Our friends Richard and Lindsay Roberts had stood in agreement with us about our conception and ability to carry the seed full term. Now, about six months into the pregnancy, Lindsay had mailed me a copy of the cassette "Supernatural Childbirth." Here I was fighting hell to conceive and carry this child, and now Lindsay and Jackie were pressing my faith a step further. I guess that's what friends are for.

To tell you all of the story of how God moved in our conception, pregnancy and delivery would make a War and Peace novel. Our God is an awesome God!

Did I have a pain-free delivery? No, I didn't. Did I have a much better delivery than I would have without "Supernatural Childbirth"? Absolutely. Do I recommend "Supernatural Childbirth" to my friends? You'd better believe it. I thank God it's now available in book form so women can study it again and again and get it deep in their spirit. I strongly suggest one for a wedding gift, so it can be seeded in before the pregnancy.

Don't expect everyone to do cartwheels when you share this revelation with them. If they don't, just smile and think the best of them. I personally think it's best to find one or two people who will stand in agreement with you and share your revelation with others after your delivery. That way, doubt and negative words can be kept at a minimum.

God has blessed us with two miracle children: Destiny, our daughter, and Israel, our son.

At age four, Destiny asked, with tears streaming down her cheeks, if she could help us pray for the sick in our prayer lines. The first woman she prayed with had cancer and had been given six months to live. Three weeks after Destiny prayed, the doctor's report showed no trace of cancer! Israel has known all the books of the Bible since he was two. I've never seen children with such pure faith and such ability to comprehend and retain the Word of God.

If you're in a battle concerning your seed, whether in your body, soul, or spirit, tighten up your combat boots!

Get yourself armed with every promise in the Word and rejoice…Children are the heritage of the Lord!

Reba Rambo McGuire
Nashville, Tennessee

9
Epilogue

by Terry Mize

When Jackie and I started to use prayer and faith to override all that doctors and family and friends had said for years and to believe God to heal Jackie's body so that we could have the family we so desired, we didn't know what we do now. Thank God we've grown and matured with each passing year and learned so much with each baby.

All we started with was prayer and God's promises to even conceive and have a healthy mommy and baby! Then we moved to being redeemed from the curse of the Law by Jesus, believing for no morning sickness, no emotional problems, no pain, no anesthetic, no stitches and so on.

We know there are two curses: the curse in the Garden and the curse of the Law. We really didn't deal much with the original curse in the Garden but with the curse of the Law in Genesis through Deuteronomy majoring on the fact that pain (any kind of pain) is under the curse of the Law and Galatians 3 says that Jesus has redeemed us from it.

One reason we didn't deal much with the curse in the Garden is that we didn't understand it all then; and now, almost three decades later, we still don't understand it all, nor do we know anyone else who does.

I've been working on a book on the subject and have done much study and have talked to countless preachers about it. One thing we do know is that the three separate and distinct curses that God placed on 1) the serpent 2) Eve and 3) Adam don't mean what the Church has always thought. The three curses brought a drastic change to the three that were cursed and their descendants, but we can't know how drastic the change because we don't know what it was like before the curse came.

This is not the time or place to go into it all; but let it suffice to say that the curse in the Garden separated God and man. God lost His relationship with man and wanted His man back, so He set in motion His plan of redemption: first, the Law and second, Jesus. Missions or soulwinning was originated in the Garden to get man back to God.

Now the word "sorrow" in Eve's curse in Genesis is the same word "sorrow" as in Adam's curse in Genesis.

> **Unto the woman he said, I will greatly multiply thy sorrow and thy conception; in SORROW thou shalt bring forth children; and thy desire shall be to thy husband, and he shall rule over thee.**

> **And unto Adam he said, Because thou hast hearkened unto the voice of thy wife, and hast eaten of the tree, of which I commanded thee, saying, Thou shalt not eat of it: cursed is the ground for thy sake; in SORROW shalt thou eat of it all the days of thy life.**
> **Genesis 3:16,17**

The Church has always wanted it to mean pain for Eve. Well, it doesn't mean pain; it means what it says, "sorrow, grief." My God did not put pain on them. He is not the author of pain. Pain, like sickness and disease, came in the package deal; it came with the curse or sin system, the beggarly elements of this world. If Eve's curse literally does mean that she will have severe pain with each conception and each birth of a baby, then it would have to mean that Adam and men must have severe pain each time they eat a meal. We know that isn't true.

What the curse does mean, what the "sorrow" does mean is that Adam and Eve and all mankind will no longer live, play, eat, and bask in the shekinah glory of God in God's Garden, in God's perfect place, in God's perfect will. No longer will all be provided by God. Now mankind will live out in the world where there are real problems, sickness, disease, inflation, recession, poverty, devils, mean people, etc. Mankind must now work for a living and must till the ground and fight weeds, insects and such. And women must have their babies in this inferior world. That is the "sorrow." I don't know about you, but it makes me sorry. I wish we were still in the Garden of Eden. But, we still have redemption through Jesus. Our faith in God's Word in the covenant of blood that Jesus gave us gives us a better quality of life. With God, it is always "according to your faith." I don't have pain when I eat, and Jackie doesn't have pain when she conceives and when she gives birth to our precious babies.

I encourage you to look for God's goodness and mercy and deliverance. Don't look for trouble or problems, and don't fight for your right to tribulate when you read the Bible.

10

Confessions and Prayers

Here are the confessions and prayers Terry wrote out and we used — many we still use today.

The Importance of Confession

I've mentioned confession or confessing the Word a number of times in this book. Let me emphasize the absolute importance of this act of faith on your part. There are over 3,000 Scriptures concerning words, mouth, tongue, lips, say and speak. Surely God must be trying to tell us something.

Confession is not new; it's as old as the Bible. It's not strange, foreign, dark or mysterious. Confession is simply agreeing out loud with God, saying what God has already said.

When we pray, we must pray the Word, and pray in agreement with God's Word. We have God's Word for every area of our life; now it's up to us to make our own words agree with God's written Word. Jesus prayed, "Not my will but Yours be done." Well, we have the will of God, the Bible. We know God's will; now we must give voice to it in our prayers and in our everyday lives.

The Bible says:

Death and life are in the power of the tongue: and they that love it shall eat the fruit thereof.

Proverbs 18:21

Thou art snared with the words of thy mouth, thou art taken with the words of thy mouth.

Proverbs 6:2

And this is the confidence that we have in him, that, if we ask any thing according to his will, he heareth us:

And if we know that he hear us, whatsoever we ask, we know that we have the petitions that we desired of him.

1 John 5:14,15

I call heaven and earth to record this day against you, that I have set before you life and death, blessing and cursing: therefore choose life, that both thou and thy seed may live.

Deuteronomy 30:19

For verily I say unto you, That whosoever shall say unto this mountain, Be thou removed, and be thou cast into the sea; and shall not doubt in his heart, but shall believe that those things which he saith shall come to pass; he shall have whatsoever he saith.

Mark 11:23

O generation of vipers, how can ye, being evil, speak good things? for out of the abundance of the heart the mouth speaketh.

Matthew 12:34

Terry and I vowed to God long ago, "We will make our words agree with Your Word in every area — marriage, children, family, health, finances, ministry — and if we don't know what Your Word says on a given subject, we won't say anything until we look it up in the Bible, then we'll say what the Bible says!"

Remember, at the first of this book I told you that "who said" is very important. Well, here is what God has said about you and your baby. Now you agree with Him.

Listed below are some Scriptures and confessions we made daily during pregnancy and some others concerning our family and ministry that we still use, pray, confess, agree with and declare and have for over two decades. In fact, if you wanted a formula or recipe for our lives and ministry, you could blend these Scriptures and confessions together, add in the Great Commission, plus the previous Scriptures I've already given you, and you would get Terry and Jackie Mize, our life and ministry.

This book of the law shall not depart out of thy mouth; but thou shalt meditate therein day and night, that thou mayest observe to do according to all that is written therein: for then thou shalt make thy way prosperous, and then thou shalt have good success.

Joshua 1:8

Then said the LORD unto me, Thou hast well seen: for I will hasten my word to perform it.

Jeremiah 1:12

I will worship toward thy holy temple, and praise thy name for thy lovingkindness and for thy truth: for thou hast magnified thy word above all thy name.

Psalm 138:2

My son, attend to my words; incline thine ear unto my sayings. Let them not depart from thine eyes; keep them in the midst of thine heart.

For they are life unto those that find them, and health to all their flesh.

Proverbs 4:20-22

It is vital that you take the Word of God and declare it from your own mouth. There is no such thing as an unimportant word or a word void of power.

I can do all things through Christ which strengtheneth me.

Philippians 4:13

But my God shall supply all your need according to his riches in glory by Christ Jesus.

Philippians 4:19

For by him were all things created, that are in heaven, and that are in earth, visible and invisible, whether they be thrones, or dominions, or principalities, or powers: all things were created by him, and for him.

Colossians 1:16

The thief cometh not, but for to steal, and to kill, and to destroy: I am come that they might have life, and that they might have it more abundantly.

John 10:10

Thou art worthy, O Lord, to receive glory and honour and power: for thou hast created all things, and for thy pleasure they are and were created.

Revelation 4:11

Being confident of this very thing, that he which hath begun a good work in you will perform it until the day of Jesus Christ.

Philippians 1:6

Let us hold fast the profession of our faith without wavering; (for he is faithful that promised.)

Hebrews 10:23

Draw nigh to God, and he will draw nigh to you. Cleanse your hands, ye sinners; and purify your hearts, ye double-minded.

James 4:8

For with God nothing shall be impossible.

Luke 1:37

Blessed is the man that walketh not in the counsel of the ungodly, nor standeth in the way of sinners, nor sitteth in the seat of the scornful.

But his delight is in the law of the LORD; and in his law doth he meditate day and night.

And he shall be like a tree planted by the rivers of water, that bringeth forth his fruit in his season; his leaf also shall not wither; and whatsoever he doeth shall prosper.

Psalm 1:1-3

And Jesus answered him, saying, It is written, That man shall not live by bread alone, but by every word of God.

Luke 4:4

How God anointed Jesus of Nazareth with the Holy Ghost and with power: who went about doing good, and healing all that were oppressed of the devil; for God was with him.

Acts 10:38

For with the heart man believeth unto righteousness; and with the mouth confession is made unto salvation.

Romans 10:10

Nay, in all these things we are more than conquerors through him that loved us.

Romans 8:37

And be not conformed to this world: but be ye transformed by the renewing of your mind, that ye may prove what is that good, and acceptable, and perfect, will of God.

Romans 12:2

Who his own self bare our sins in his own body on the tree, that we, being dead to sins, should live unto righteousness: by whose stripes ye were healed.

1 Peter 2:24

Give, and it shall be given unto you; good measure, pressed down, and shaken together, and running over, shall men give into your bosom. For with the same measure that ye mete withal it shall be measured to you again.

Luke 6:38

Bring ye all the tithes into the storehouse, that there may be meat in mine house, and prove me now herewith, saith the LORD of hosts, if I will not open you the windows of heaven, and pour you out a blessing, that there shall not be room enough to receive it.

And I will rebuke the devourer for your sakes, and he shall not destroy the fruits of your ground; neither shall your vine cast her fruit before the time in the field, saith the LORD of hosts.

Malachi 3:10,11

Beloved, I wish above all things that thou mayest prosper and be in health, even as thy soul prospereth.

3 John 2

Surely he hath borne our griefs, and carried our sorrows: yet we did esteem him stricken, smitten of God, and afflicted.

But he was wounded for our transgressions, he was bruised for our iniquities: the chastisement of our peace was upon him; and with his stripes we are healed.

Isaiah 53:4,5

And all thy children shall be taught of the LORD; and great shall be the peace of thy children.

In righteousness shalt thou be established: thou shalt be far from oppression; for thou shalt not fear: and from terror; for it shall not come near thee.

Behold, they shall surely gather together, but not by me: whosoever shall gather together against thee shall fall for thy sake.

Isaiah 54:13-15

No weapon that is formed against thee shall prosper; and every tongue that shall rise against thee in judgment thou shalt condemn. This is the heritage of the servants of the LORD, and their righteousness is of me, saith the LORD.

Isaiah 54:17

Use the following verses from Galatians to negate the curses of the Law found especially in Deuteronomy chapter 28.

Christ hath redeemed us from the curse of the law, being made a curse for us: for it is written, Cursed is every one that hangeth on a tree:

That the blessing of Abraham might come on the Gentiles through Jesus Christ; that we might receive the promise of the Spirit through faith.

And if ye be Christ's, then are ye Abraham's seed, and heirs according to the promise.

Galatians 3:13,14,29

Now don't forget the Great Commission found in Matthew 28:19,20; Mark 16:15-18; Luke 24:47; John 20:21; and Acts 1:8.

Dealing With Fear and Thoughts

Fear is a spiritual force. It is the opposite of faith. Fear is real, and it is not of God. It affects the life we live on planet earth. It affects the physical body. It can put a wrinkle in the skin, change the color of hair, make the heart beat fast or even stop. It has killed many people over the years. The Bible says in the last days men's hearts will fail them for fear. (Luke 21:26.) Fear motivates Satan as faith motivates God. Fear is Satan's tool as faith is God's.

You only fear the unknown or past bad experiences. Past failures bring future fears. Fear and faith don't operate together. Fear is your worst enemy when it's allowed to operate. It can be one of the greatest causes of pain during childbirth.

Now don't get scared. I've got good news for you. Actually, the Word of God has good news for you. The Bible says in 1 John 4:18 that fear has torment but perfect love casts out fear. Now, God is love (1 John 4:16) the Bible says, and you've got God, so fear must go.

Second Timothy 1:7 says: **For God hath not given us the spirit of fear; but of power, and of love, and of a sound mind.** You can conquer fear in Jesus' name with faith in God's Word. And Romans 10:17 says, **So then faith cometh by hearing, and hearing by the word of God.**

All through the Bible God says "Fear not...." "Don't be afraid...." Doesn't it make sense that when you are at peace, your body will be relaxed; it can stretch more, be more elastic? On the other hand, fear causes your body and muscles and nerves to tense up, to tighten. Jesus said, "My peace I leave with you." (John 14:27.) Faith in God's Word brings peace.

F - alse
E - vidence
A - bout
R - eality

Prayer/Confession

Father, I come before You in the mighty name of Jesus and the covenant of blood, and I rebuke fear and doubt and unbelief. Your Word says You have not given me a spirit of fear but of love and power and of a sound mind. Your Word also says that fear has torment but that perfect love casts out fear and that God is love, and I've got God living big in me so fear and torment go far from me now in Jesus' name. I trust in the Lord; I will not fear; I will not be afraid. I have the mind of Christ and the peace of God. My mind and body, as well as my spirit, are relaxed and at peace. I refuse to let my heart be troubled or afraid.

The Lord, Most High, is my light and my salvation, whom shall I fear? The Lord, El Shaddi, is the strength of my life, of whom shall I be afraid?

Body, I speak to you to be at peace, relax, rest. Muscles, nerves, be at peace. I rest in faith in God's Word and thank You, Father, for total and complete peace and confidence, in Jesus' name, Amen.

Ps. 112:7; Isa. 41:10; Ps.27:1; Isa.54:17; John 14:27; 1 John 4:18; Phil. 4:7,8; Eph. 4:27; Isa.26:3; 1 Peter 5:7

HERE ARE SOME MORE SCRIPTURES FOR YOU TO THINK ON AND TO CONFESS.

When thou liest down, thou shalt not be afraid: yea, thou shalt lie down, and thy sleep shall be sweet.

Proverbs 3:24

I sought the LORD, and he heard me, and delivered me from all my fears.

Psalm 34:4

And to you who are troubled rest with us, when the Lord Jesus shall be revealed from heaven with his mighty angels.

2 Thessalonians 1:7

Casting down imaginations, and every high thing that exalteth itself against the knowledge of God, and bringing into captivity every thought to the obedience of Christ.

2 Corinthians 10:5

No weapon that is formed against thee shall prosper; and every tongue that shall rise against thee in judgment thou shalt condemn. This is the heritage of the servants of the LORD, and their righteousness is of me, saith the LORD.

Isaiah 54:17

He sent his word, and healed them, and delivered them from their destructions.

Psalm 107:20

Let us therefore come boldly unto the throne of grace, that we may obtain mercy, and find grace to help in time of need.

Hebrews 4:16

And be not conformed to this world: but be ye transformed by the renewing of your mind, that ye may prove what is that good, and acceptable, and perfect, will of God.

Romans 12:2

For I know the thoughts that I think toward you, saith the Lord, thoughts of peace, and not of evil, to give you an expected end.

Jeremiah 29:11

Delight thyself also in the Lord; and he shall give thee the desires of thine heart.

Psalm 37:4

Confession: Psalm 91

I don't know of a more effective confession in the Bible than Psalm 91. We confess this on a daily basis. The keys to making Psalm 91 work for you are found in verses 1 and 2. You must be dwelling in the secret place of the Most High, abiding in the shadow of the Almighty. How do you do that? Verse 2 tells you: You must "Say of the Lord."

We pray it like this:

"Father, we thank You that we (our family, our ministry) dwell in the secret place of the Most High, and we abide under the shadow of the Almighty. For we boldly say, decree and declare that the Lord, El Shaddi, the God Who is more than enough, Jehovah Jireh, Jehovah Rapha, Jehovah Tsidkenu, Jehovah Shalom, Jehovah Nissi, Jehovah Rapha, Jehovah Shammah, the possessor of heaven and earth, is our God. We trust in Him — some trust in horses, some in chariots, but we trust in the name of the Lord our God. He is our refuge and our fortress, our God, in Him do we trust. Surely He shall deliver us from the snare of the fowler and from the noisome pestilence. He shall cover us with His feathers, and under His wings shall we trust; His truth shall be our shield and buckler. We shall not be afraid for the terror by night, nor for the arrow that flieth by day, nor for the pestilence that walketh in darkness, nor for the destruction that wasteth at noonday. A thousand shall fall at our side and ten thousand at our right hand, but it shall not come nigh us. Only with our eyes shall we behold and see the reward of the wicked.

"Because we have made the Lord which is our refuge, even the Most High, our habitation, there shall no evil befall us, neither shall any plague come nigh our dwelling. For He shall give His angels charge over us, to keep us in all our ways. They shall bear us up in their hands lest we dash our foot against a stone. We shall tread upon the lion and the adder; the young lion and the dragon shall we trample under foot.

"Because we have set our love upon Him; therefore, will He deliver us. He will set us on high, because we have known His name. We shall call upon Him, and He will answer us. He will be with us in trouble; He will deliver us and honor us. With long life will He satisfy us and show us His salvation. Salvation is of the Lord. In Jesus' name."

Ps. 91:1-16; Ps. 20:7

Confession: Psalm 103

"Father, according to Psalm 103 I say, **Bless the LORD, O my soul: and all that is within me, bless his holy name. Bless the LORD, O my soul, and forget not all his benefits.** I say it and decree it over our family and our ministry and all that our family has anything to do with. I declare that those benefits belong to us. We'll not forget the benefits of the Lord: that our iniquities are forgiven, every sin is under the blood of Jesus. Father, Your Word says that if we confess our sins, You are faithful and just to forgive us our sins and to cleanse us from all unrighteousness. So we put every thought, every deed that's wrong, that is not pleasing to You under the blood of Jesus. We ask forgiveness, Lord. And we say that we are cleansed and forgiven in Jesus' name. Father, we thank You for that.

"We say that You redeem our lives from destruction. We are protected by You, by Your Word, by Your angels. We'll not die prematurely; we'll not be destroyed. The destroyer, the accuser of the brethren, has been cast down. We're redeemed from destruction. Our lives will not be destroyed.

"You heal all our diseases. You crown us with lovingkindness and tender mercies. You satisfy our mouth with good things. I say that we have good things to speak and good things to eat so that our youth is renewed like the eagles. We'll not be old, decrepit and senile; even though we gain in age, we'll not go downhill. We wait on the Lord, and our youth is renewed.

"Bless the Lord, O my soul, and all that is within me, bless His holy name. We thank You for all those benefits, and we'll be careful not to forget them. We give You glory and honor and thanks in Jesus' name."

Ps. 103:1-5; 1 John 1:9

Before Pregnancy: Desire To Conceive, Fulfillment Over Barrenness

"Father, we thank You that children are the heritage of the Lord, and the fruit of the womb is His reward. Children are Your idea Father; You thought up children, and family and home. You instituted the family in the Garden of Eden. You ordered children; You commanded them when You said to Adam and Eve, 'Be fruitful and multiply.' You said that the barren womb is never satisfied. Lord, the Word declares that I am wonderfully and fearfully made by You; therefore, I'm perfect and able to conceive and have children. You said that I/(my wife) would be a fruitful vine by the side of our house and our children like olive plants around our table. We are not ashamed but happy because our quiver is full of children (or arrows, as You call them).

"Thank You, Father, that You designed and fashioned me/her, to have children, that in the Bible barrenness was the exception, not the rule, not Your will, not normal, something against Your plan and purpose. And in Your goodness and faithfulness, every barren woman in the Bible who was godly and believed Your Word became pregnant; You opened her womb and blessed her, and she gave birth to a precious baby just as I/she will. You make the barren woman to keep house and to be a joyful mother of children.

"You said, Father, that because You are our God and we are Your people and have a covenant with You, that You will love us and bless us and multiply us and bless the fruit of my/her womb and that neither male nor female among Your people would be barren.

"Father, we are redeemed from the curse of the Law by Jesus and being barren is under the curse of the Law;

therefore, we will receive from Your grace and have children.

"Father, no plague, no evil shall come nigh our dwelling. We are healed by the stripes of Jesus. Sickness of any kind is taken out of our midst. You said to ask anything of You in Jesus' name and it would be done; and that if two of us on earth agree as touching anything it would be done. So we pray and we agree with You and Your Word, Father, that we will conceive and bring forth a healthy, precious baby to Your glory and honor. We pray all this according to Your Word and will. You said, This is the confidence that we have in You, that if we ask anything according to Your will, You hear us; and if You hear us, we know we have the petition we desire of You. We have it now. Thank You, Father, in Jesus' name."

Ps. 127:3; Gen. 1:28; Ps. 139:14; Ps. 128:3; Ps. 127:4,5; Ps. 113:9; Gal. 3:13; Ps. 91; 1 Peter 2:24; Ex. 23:25; John 16:23; Matt. 18:19; 1 John 5:14,15.

NOW, TALK TO YOUR BODY:

"Body, we speak to you in Jesus' name: You will come in line and agreement with the Word of God. You will respond to His holy Word. You will function properly and perfectly, the way God intended you to. Every part, every organ of our reproductive system conforms to the Word and plan of God as we come together in pure, marital love. Body, conceive! Be pregnant. Cooperate with God's plan: perfect ovulation, release of perfect eggs from the ovaries, through the fallopian tubes, penetrated and impregnated, fertilized by healthy sperm. Good solid attachment to uterine wall and nourished and protected for nine months (40 weeks) unharmed and unhindered. Grow to a perfect baby — spirit, soul and body. Your Word says, Father, that none shall cast their young, nor be barren among Your people and the number of our days You will fulfill. This pregnancy will be fulfilled. We decree it in Jesus' name and receive God's best; we won't settle for anything less in Jesus' holy name. Thank You, Lord, that it is so and done to Your honor and glory. Amen."

Ex. 23:26

Now at this point — before conception — is the proper time to build your faith. Don't wait; do it now. Listen to my tape every day or two.[1] Get this book and these Scriptures and truths in your spirit until they are real to you, until you are thinking them and talking them and believing them.

If you want a particular sex in this baby, now is the time to believe for that — not after conception.

If you want a boy or if you want a girl, set your faith early — set it now. Ask God for the desire of your heart.

If you know of a problem in your body, a deficiency or malfunction, now is the time to believe for your healing. Get ready physically to get pregnant.

Speak to your body every day to conceive, carry and deliver your baby. Do it in faith; don't do it in fear.

These "barren" women "conceived and bare" children. You set your faith to conceive and bare also, in Jesus' name.

Sarah

But Sarai was barren; she had no child...

And he said, I will certainly return unto thee according to the time of life; and, lo, Sarah thy wife shall have a son. And Sarah heard it in the tent door, which was behind him.

Now Abraham and Sarah were old and well stricken in age; and it ceased to be with Sarah after the manner of women...

---

[1]You can order my tape, "Supernatural Childbirth," from me at the address in the back of the book. Cost is $7.00 + $2.00 shipping and handling.

And the Lord visited Sarah as he had said, and the Lord did unto Sarah as he had spoken.

For Sarah conceived, and bare Abraham a son in his old age, at the set time of which God had spoken to him.

Genesis 11:30; 18:10,11; 21:1,2

Rebekah

And Isaac entreated the Lord for his wife, because she was barren: and the Lord was entreated of him, and Rebekah his wife conceived.

Genesis 25:21

Leah

And when the Lord saw that Leah was hated, he opened her womb: but Rachel was barren.

Genesis 29:31

Rachel

And when Rachel saw that she bare Jacob no children, Rachel envied her sister; and said unto Jacob, Give me children, or else I die...

And God remembered Rachel, and God hearkened to her, and opened her womb.

And she conceived, and bare a son; and said, God hath taken away my reproach.

Genesis 30:1,22,23

Hannah

For this child I prayed; and the Lord hath given me my petition which I asked of him.

1 Samuel 1:27

Manoah's wife, Samson's mother

And there was a certain man of Zorah, of the family of the Danites, whose name was Manoah; and his wife was barren, and bare not.

And the angel of the Lord appeared unto the woman, and said unto her, Behold now, thou art barren, and barest not: but thou shalt conceive, and bear a son.

And the woman bare a son, and called his name Samson: and the child grew, and the Lord blessed him.

Judges 13:2,3,24

Ruth

We don't know if Ruth was barren, but she didn't have children with her first husband. She did, however, become the great-grandmother of David.

So Boaz took Ruth, and she was his wife: and when he went in unto her, the Lord gave her conception, and she bare a son.

Ruth 4:13

Shunammite Woman

And he said, What then is to be done for her? And Gehazi answered, Verily she hath no child, and her husband is old.

And he said, Call her. And when he had called her, she stood in the door.

And the woman conceived, and bare a son at that season that Elisha had said unto her, according to the time of life.

2 Kings 4:14,15,17

Elisabeth, mother of John the Baptist

And they had no child, because that Elisabeth was barren, and they both were now well stricken in years...

And after those days his wife Elisabeth conceived, and hid herself five months, saying,

Thus hath the Lord dealt with me in the days wherein he looked on me, to take away my reproach among men.

Luke 1:7,24,25

THESE ARE GOOD SCRIPTURES FOR PRAYERS AND CONFESSIONS

And he will love thee, and bless thee, and multiply thee: he will also bless the fruit of thy womb, and the fruit of thy land, thy corn, and thy wine, and thine oil, the increase of thy kine, and the flocks of thy sheep, in the land which he sware unto thy fathers to give thee.

Thou shalt be blessed above all people: there shall not be male or female barren among you, or among your cattle.

And the Lord will take away from thee all sickness, and will put none of the evil diseases of Egypt, which thou knowest, upon thee; but will lay them upon all them that hate thee.

Deuteronomy 7:13-15

And ye shall serve the Lord your God, and he shall bless thy bread, and thy water; and I will take sickness away from the midst of thee.

There shall nothing cast their young, nor be barren, in thy land: the number of thy days I will fulfill.

Exodus 23:25,26

There shall no evil befall thee, neither shall any plague come nigh thy dwelling.

Psalm 91:10

He maketh the barren woman to keep house, and to be a joyful mother of children. Praise ye the Lord.

Psalm 113:9

Lo, children are an heritage of the Lord: and the fruit of the womb is his reward.

As arrows are in the hand of a mighty man; so are children of the youth.

Happy is the man that hath his quiver full of them: they shall not be ashamed, but they shall speak with the enemies in the gate.

Psalm 127:3-5

Thy wife shall be as a fruitful vine by the sides of thine house: thy children like olive plants round about thy table.

Psalm 128:3

During Pregnancy or Threatening Miscarriage

You don't find "miscarriage" or "abortion" in the Bible. It was not and is not today the will of God for you to lose your baby. God wants you and your baby healthy, whole and prosperous spiritually, physically, mentally, and financially. God is a good God.

There are multitudes of Scriptures you can pray and confess during this time, but these are good and will get you started. Use these Scriptures and the following prayer/confession all the time you are pregnant.

> And ye shall serve the Lord your God, and he shall bless thy bread, and thy water; and I will take sickness away from the midst of thee.
>
> There shall nothing cast their young, nor be barren, in thy land: the number of thy days I will fulfil.
>
> **Exodus 23:25,26**

> And he will love thee, and bless thee, and multiply thee: he will also bless the fruit of thy womb, and the fruit of thy land, thy corn, and thy wine, and thine oil, the increase of thy kine, and the flocks of thy sheep, in the land which he sware unto thy fathers to give thee.
>
> **Deuteronomy 7:13**

> Bring ye all the tithes into the storehouse, that there may be meat in mine house, and prove me now herewith, saith the Lord of hosts, if I will not open you the windows of heaven, and pour you out a blessing, that there shall not be room enough to receive it.
>
> And I will rebuke the devourer for your sakes, and he shall not destroy the fruits of your ground; neither shall your vine cast her fruit before the time in the field.
>
> **Malachi 3:10,11**

Just as I said to you that all barren women in the Bible conceived, I want you to know that every woman in the Bible that conceived gave birth, she had her baby, and she and the baby were healthy. There are two notable exceptions.

In Genesis 35, Rachel, wife of Jacob, had hard labor and died while giving birth. She is the only one in the Bible that it particularly points out a different pattern — hard labor, the exception, not the rule. She had stolen some images of gods from Laban (her father). Her husband, Jacob, not knowing that she had stolen them, made a decree that whoever had stolen them would die. She did.

Bathsheba and David's baby died of sickness seven days after he was born. You can read this in 2 Samuel chapters 11 and 12. David had taken Bathsheba in adultery, and she conceived. David then had her husband killed and took her for his own wife. God sent Nathan the prophet to tell David that he would not die but the baby would.

You do find in the Bible that babies, even in the womb (uterus), were real and alive and known to God. This should answer any and all questions about abortion and "when is the fetus alive."

Luke 1:41 says of John the Baptist,

And it came to pass, that, when Elisabeth heard the salutation of Mary, the babe leaped in her womb; and Elisabeth was filled with the Holy Ghost.

In Genesis 25:23 God told Rebekah of her boys in her womb that,

Two nations are in thy womb, and two manner of people shall be separated from thy bowels; and the one people shall be stronger than the other people; and the elder shall serve the younger.

God didn't just see "fetuses"; He saw men and the nations they would become.

In Judges 13:5,7, God said that Samson was a Nazarite from the womb to the day of his death.

For thou hast possessed my reins: thou hast covered me in my mother's womb.

Psalm 139:13

Thus saith the Lord that made thee, and formed thee from the womb, which will help thee; Fear not, O Jacob, my servant; and thou, Jesurun, whom I have chosen.

Isaiah 44:2

But when it pleased God, who separated me from my mother's womb, and called me by his grace.

Galatians 1:15

Before I formed thee in the belly I knew thee; and before thou camest forth out of the womb I sanctified thee, and I ordained thee a prophet unto the nations.

Jeremiah 1:5

Prayer/Confession

"Thank You, Father, for this child. I can say with Hannah, 'For this child I prayed and the Lord hath given me my petition which I asked of him.'

"Thank You, Lord, for a wonderful pregnancy, an enjoyable pregnancy. Thank You that I am in control over my body and the Word has preeminence in my life. I will not be subject to my emotions, but they are subject to Your Word. I'll not have morning sickness. You said You bless my bread and water and take sickness out of my midst. Not only will I enjoy this pregnancy, but my family will, as well. It will be a good time, a pleasant time. I'll rest well and sleep well. You said You give Your beloved sleep. I'll watch what I eat and not gain too much weight. The children of Israel walked forty years in the wilderness and their feet didn't swell; my feet will not swell in Jesus' name. Thank You for what Your Word calls blessings of the breasts and of the womb (Gen. 49:25). I'll not have sore or cracked nipples and breasts.

"I will feel and be feminine. I radiate life. I glow and am attractive during this pregnancy. My husband and children will enjoy being with me, and I will enjoy being with them. I'll be amorous and loving toward my husband. Your Word says that he is always ravished with my love and my breasts satisfy him at all times. He has no need of spoil during this time and he drinks waters out of his own well, and he rejoices with the wife of his youth, the wife of his covenant — me! We will continue to have a good and blessed sex life during this pregnancy!

"This pregnancy will be full duration, full term. I'm a tither, and my vine won't cast its fruit before its time in the field. You said I would not cast my young or miscarry and the number of my days You would fulfill. Thank You that You bless the fruit of my womb. My baby is covered in my womb as David declared. You said numerous times in the Bible that You formed and fashioned our baby in the womb and at the right time You will separate my baby from my womb and carry it gently from my womb.

"Father, I declare over this precious one, as I do over all my family, that we are healed by the stripes of Jesus. No sickness, no plague, no evil can come upon us. Your angels have charge over us and keep us in all our ways and lift us up lest we dash our foot against a stone. Just like all the ladies of faith in the Bible, I will give birth to a healthy, whole baby, a child whose heart is toward God and Your promise. And Your command is that if we train this child up in the way he/she should go that he/she won't depart from it when he/she is old. Our baby will honor his/her father and mother and obey; therefore, it will be well (not sick) with our child, and he/she will live long on the earth.

"Father, I speak to my body and to my baby — to every part, every organ, every system to function properly and perfectly, fully developed as You intended from the beginning. I declare health, wholeness, soundness, spirit, soul, and body from the top of the head to the bottom of the feet."

Speak to your baby in the womb. It's your baby and is supposed to obey you and God's Word.

NOTE: At this point, you can be as specific as you want to be. If you know of a problem in your family (heredity, sickness) you can address that. The important thing is that you are agreeing in faith with God and His Word, not just babbling out of fear. The concept of confession is not begging or pleading with God but thanking and agreeing with Him.

We spoke to many areas or as many as we could think of:

Eyes: Vision, be perfect. (Moses was 120 years old and his eye wasn't dim.)

Ears: Hear perfectly.

Skin: Complexion, be good.

Teeth: Form perfectly. Be strong, not prone to cavities. (Song of Solomon 4:2; 6:6.)

Bones: Be strong, healthy, straight, none broken. (Ps. 34:20.)

Heart: Be strong, healthy, untroubled. (John 14:1.)

Respiratory system: Be healthy and strong lungs and bronchial passages; no sinus problems, hay fever, bronchitis.

Blood: Be normal, healthy. Maintain the proper blood sugar; no pollution in the blood. (Ezek. 16:6.)

Digestive system: Function normally.

Position of baby and cord: Baby, be head down and in perfect position at birth. Cord, be the perfect length and position, not around the baby's neck.

Temperament: Be full of peace — a calm, sweet spirit and a tender heart. (Isa. 54:13.)

Sleeping habits: Baby, you will sleep at night; you will get plenty of rest and let us rest.

Baby's spirit: You will be tender toward God and the things of God; saved at an early age.

If parents or grandparents have a physical problem, DON'T confess that on your baby. Don't say, "It will have grandfather's teeth" or an aunt's complexion or any family member's problems. But mirror God's Word to Him. Say to God and to you and to your mate and to your baby what God has already said, what God has already willed and written.

Finish the confession:

"We pray for the medical professionals we are involved with that they have the mind of Christ and wisdom of God concerning our family and this baby. The eyes of their understanding be opened that You, Father, lead and guide them how to care for me/my wife by Your Spirit. I say we have favor with them, that they are cooperative with us and what we are doing, that all is well and peaceful and under control in Jesus' name."

"Thank You, Father, for this time for our family and time to spend with You. Thank You for fulfilling Your promise in Your Word. In Jesus' name. Amen."

1 Sam. 1:27; Ex. 23:25; Ps. 127:2; Deut. 8:4; Gen. 49:25; Prov. 5:19; Prov. 5:15; Mal. 3:11; Ex. 23:26; Deut. 7:13; Ps. 139:13; Isa. 44:2; Gal. 1:15; Jer. 1:5; Ps. 71:6; Ps. 22:9,10; 1 Peter 2:24; Ps. 91:10-12; Prov. 22:6; Eph. 6:2,3; 3 John 2; Ezek. 16:6; Isa. 54:13; Eph. 1:17,18; Prov. 3:3,4.

Delivery

"Father, as I look forward to delivery of my sweet baby, having enjoyed a blessed pregnancy of full duration, I thank You in advance for Your Word, Your blessings, Your peace, Your presence and Your divine intervention. I pray and confess that my body and my baby will cooperate with perfect, supernatural delivery, that there will be no problems of any kind. I also believe and declare that my labor and delivery will be quick, short, easy and painless. I believe and declare that I'll have time to get to the proper place with the proper help.

"Baby, in Jesus' name, you move and place yourself in perfect position for birth: head first, not breech and face down. You rotate properly as God intended you to. I command the umbilical cord to be in proper position as well. Body, you function perfectly during this time. I have perfect peace and am relaxed. All fear must go and stay gone for I have God, Who is perfect love and casts out fear. My body will not be tense but relaxed, at peace. I speak specifically to all the parts of my body to come in line with God's Word and will.

"Father, I believe that at the proper time for delivery my water will break and my uterus will do its job and begin to contract and push my baby down the birth canal and out into our loving arms and lives. I command my cervix to dilate fully to 10 cm., to be elastic and stretch. To the uterus, vagina, perineum, vulva as well as my cervix, you relax, be elastic and stretch without causing pain or any complications. Accommodate the birth of my baby. Furthermore, I declare in Jesus' name that I will not tear or need an episiotomy. Father, pain is under the curse of the Law, and Your Word says that Jesus bore our pain, so I rebuke all pain and will not tolerate pain. I will have a short, easy, pain free delivery in Jesus' name; therefore, I won't need any anesthetic of any kind. Thank You, Lord, in Jesus' name. Amen."

Ex. 1:19; 1 John 4:16; 1 John 4:18; Matt. 8:17; Deut. 28

Baby Dedication

We believe in presenting babies in solemn dedication to God. We see in the Bible that parents brought children to Jesus for His blessing. (Matt. 19:13-15; Mark 10:13-16.) Jesus put His hands on them and blessed them.

Hannah brought baby Samuel to church and presented him to God. (1 Sam. 1:22-28.) And Joseph and Mary brought baby Jesus to church and presented Him to God. (Luke 2:22-24.)

Terry and I, as ministers, have been brought babies by the multitudes of parents and in some nations, we have not only had the job of dedicating the baby through prayer to God but of naming the child as well.

We have prayed over and dedicated our four children in formal church services with congregations as witnesses and also privately both before conception and while the baby was in the womb.

Realize that "Baby Dedication" is your presentation of your child to God forever: that God be first and foremost in the child's life; that God use your child for His will; that God protect and provide for your child spirit, soul and body; that you understand that your child is God's and is only on loan to you, that you cannot just do as you please with your child but you have commandments and instructions in the Bible on how to rear and treat your child.

God said of Abraham, "I know him. He will command his children in the ways of God." (Gen. 18:19.)

Remember, just because you give your baby back to God, He still expects and commands you to raise him and care for him on earth.

Here is a prayer you can adapt or pray as it is both privately, just you and God, or before a minister in church.

"Father, in Jesus' holy name, we come before You on this special day to present to You, to consecrate to You, to dedicate to You, to give back to You, this, our sweet baby that You have given us. Lord, we realize that we are only stewards of this special gift from You. Only You create life. This baby is Your baby. You said I must teach my children of You and Your commandments. You promised that if we would train up our child in the way he should go he would not depart from it when he is old. You promised that if children would honor their parents it would be well with them (not sick but well) and they would live long on the earth. You said they would be disciples of the Lord, taught and obedient to the Lord and great would be their peace and undisturbed composure. Thank You for these promises and commandments. Thank You for our baby.

"This day, before You and the host of heaven and all other witnesses, we come to present to You in solemn dedication our baby. We consecrate as parents to not provoke him to wrath, but to bring him up in the nurture and admonition of the Lord. We commit to You to train him up in Your ways and he won't depart from them. We promise to teach him of You, Your ways, Your Word, Your will. We promise to train him by example and demonstration as well as our words. We promise to discipline him according to Your Word. We promise to love and care for him and bathe him in prayer from this day forward. We commit this baby into Your care. You can be omnipresent; I can't always be there, but You can. Your angels have charge over him to keep him in all his ways and lift him up lest he dash his foot against a stone. We pray that this child be healthy, whole, complete, blessed and prosperous spirit, soul and body. We bind the forces of hell and the devil in Jesus' name to stay away from our family in every area of our lives. We decree that Jesus be enthroned above all else in our family at all times in Jesus' name. Amen."

Deut. 6:6,7; Prov. 22:6; Eph. 6:1-3; Isa. 54:13; Eph. 6:4; Prov. 22:15; Prov. 29:15; Ps. 91

Salvation Prayer

God loves you—no matter who you are, no matter what your past. God loves you so much that He gave His one and only begotten Son for you. The Bible tells us that "...whoever believes in him shall not perish but have eternal life" (John 3:16 NIV). Jesus laid down His life and rose again so that we could spend eternity with Him in heaven and experience His absolute best on earth. If you would like to receive Jesus into your life, say the following prayer out loud and mean it from your heart.

Heavenly Father, I come to You admitting that I am a sinner. Right now, I choose to turn away from sin, and I ask You to cleanse me of all unrighteousness. I believe that Your Son, Jesus, died on the cross to take away my sins. I also believe that He rose again from the dead so that I might be forgiven of my sins and made righteous through faith in Him. I call upon the name of Jesus Christ to be the Savior and Lord of my life. Jesus, I choose to follow You and ask that You fill me with the power of the Holy Spirit. I declare that right now I am a child of God. I am free from sin and full of the righteousness of God. I am saved in Jesus' name. Amen

If you prayed this prayer to receive Jesus Christ as your Savior for the first time, please contact us on the web at www.harrisonhouse.com to receive a free book.

Or you may write to us at
Harrison House Publishers
P.O. Box 35035
Tulsa, Oklahoma 74153

Terry and Jackie Mize, missionaries for over twenty years, have maintained that delicate balance of staying in line with God's priorities and fulfilling, effectively, His call on their lives to the ministry.

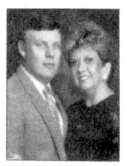

Traveling throughout the continents, ministering in open-air crusades, pastors' conferences, Bible school seminars, and church meetings, on an average of every other month in foreign countries, Terry and Jackie have made the effort necessary to take the children with them. From crusades in Mexico to Bible schools in Australia, the children attend the meetings adding their faith and support to the ministry.

In a crusade in India during which the entire family had attended two four-hour day sessions each day, and then a very long crusade each night, there is video footage of Cristy Denise, then eight years old, sleeping during the praise service and her daddy's sermon, and waking up just in time to watch the miracles — every night! They never tire of seeing the wonderful works of God.

Terry, a founding member of the Board of Trustees and chairman of the Missions Committee of the International Convention of Faith Ministries, founding board member of Victory World Missions Training Center, and Jackie, with many demands on their time, have devoted themselves, with their children, to give Living Bread to dying men around the world.

To contact the author, write: Jackie Mize
Terry Mize Ministries
P.O. Box 35044
Tulsa, OK 74153

Additional copies of this book available
at www.harrisonhouse.com

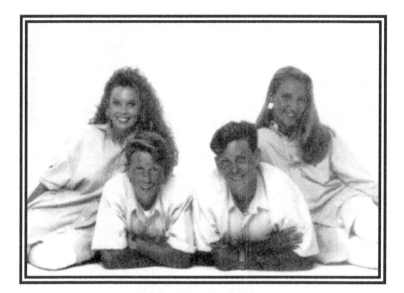

Lori Dawn, Paul David,
Lynn Noel, and Cristy Denise Mize
(left to right)

Paul David

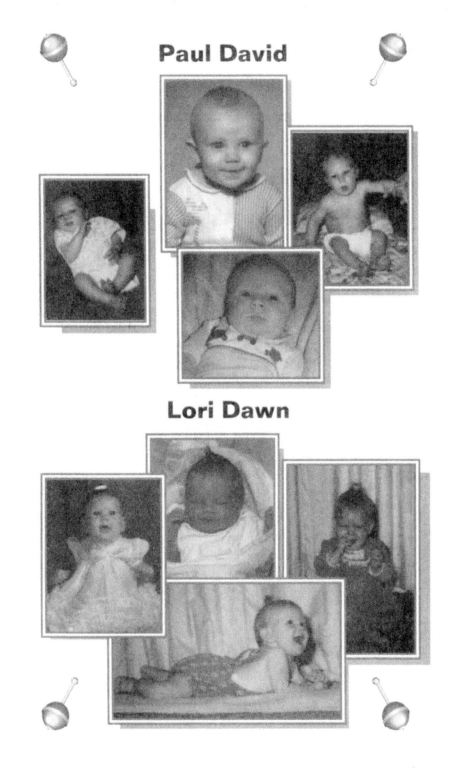

Lori Dawn

Lynn Noel

Cristy Denise

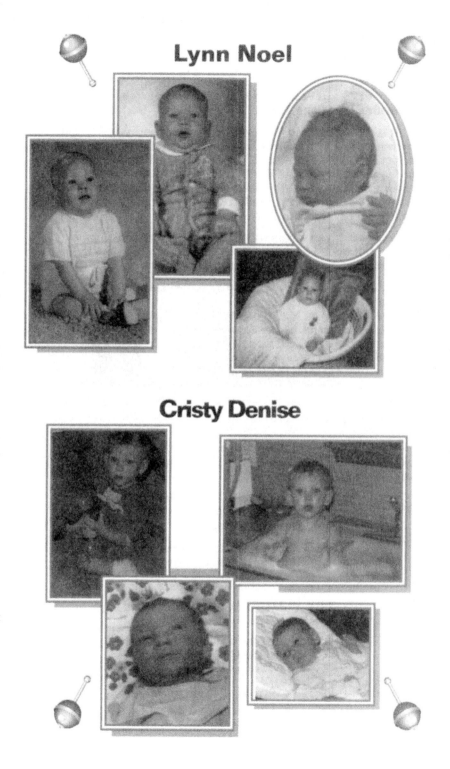

Fast. Easy.
Convenient.

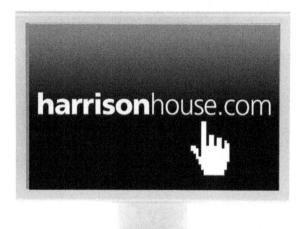

For the latest Harrison House product information and author news, look no further than your computer. All the details on our powerful, life-changing products are just a click away. New releases, E-mail subscriptions, Podcasts, testimonies, monthly specials—find it all in one place. Visit harrisonhouse.com today!

harrisonhouse

Made in the USA
Las Vegas, NV
10 January 2022